# FINDING MEANING IN WORK
## THE MUSINGS OF A TRUE GENERALIST

## WJ CRUMP

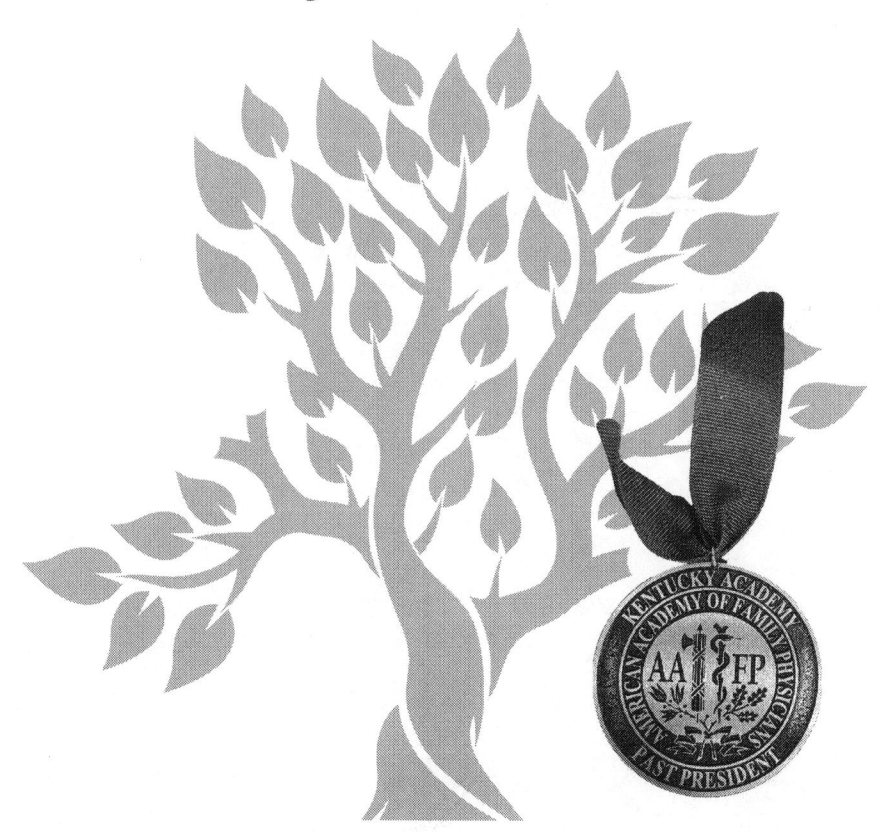

*Finding Meaning in Work: The Musings of a True Generalist*
Copyright © 2023 by WJ Crump
All rights reserved.

First Edition: 2023

No part of this book may be reproduced, scanned, or distributed in any printed or electronic form without permission. Please do not participate in or encourage piracy of copyrighted materials in violation of the author's rights. Thank you for respecting the hard work of this author.

*This book is dedicated to my parents who always made clear that they were proud of me, each in their own way. I also wish to acknowledge the many patients, teachers, and colleagues who travelled this road with me. I express my sincere thanks and undying love for my family, especially my wife Vanessa who always tolerated and supported my eccentricities. I couldn't have done it without you.*

# SYMBOLISM OF THE COVER

The accomplishments of a long medical career are often symbolized by the awards received, like a medal for a race well-run or a badge of recognition granted by one's peers. These are summative accolades that signify an end and carry an air of perfection. To the author the oak tree in his back yard is a more fitting symbol. Long the representation of spiritual wisdom back to the days of the Druids, the mighty oak speaks of the continuing process of nature. Leaves sprout each spring and find their way back to the earth each fall. New branches form, some are lost to the wind, and the central structure abides. This particular tree bears the crescent of damage from a severe ice storm that took down many less strongly rooted trees. Like the author's work, it is not perfect, but heals a bit more each year.

# FAMILY PERSPECTIVE

This book is a compilation of the author's professional work. Seamlessly interwoven across these forty years was a home life that was his central focus. Each year in his family Thanksgiving prayer, he reminded himself and all gathered around his table the priority of importance: Faith, Family, Food, and Football. The book begins with his poem of thanks for his father and here are recorded some perspectives from his family on his work life.

**Sister**

I've had the good fortune throughout the years to have my brother share with me highlights of his full and most interesting career and many of his writings. Early on, his work on the international space station in Huntsville, Alabama both puzzled and fascinated me. How was a family practice doc selected for this assignment and what could he possibly contribute? Little did I know… After he and his family moved to Galveston, TX, I learned he was testing and proving a method for physicians to reach out to people in far flung rural communities by "computer" to actually perform medical assessments and provide much needed treatment. I was, at the very best, "doubtful". Thus was the birth of telehealth! I learned of many of these professional accomplishments through the writings he authored and shared with me. Those writings kept me up at night trying to fathom the many experiences he described. The free medical clinic for the financially disadvantaged and medically underserved population he established and the mentoring he provided while recruiting medical students to staff it was a proud moment for me. In more recent years, he and his wife have welcomed medically fragile infants into their home and cared for them as they did their own children. Why am I so proud of Dr. Crump? He is my "baby brother" who continues to inspire me with his knowledge, medical skills, insightful understanding of human nature and, above all, sincere empathy for everyone in need of his help.

## Wife

When I reflect on my husband's career, the one word that comes to mind is diverse. When we met during his residency, I thought I was marrying a family physician who loved delivering babies. That turned out to be only part of the story. His opportunities with space station design brought truly unique interactions into our home. During a visit, a young Russian life support scientist still active in the party got into a fairly heated argument with a visiting older family member about Stalin's legacy. Our other Russian visitors, when not provoked, were ideal guests and their stories were much appreciated by our children. As my husband taught at International Space University, I had to explain to our children the lifestyle of those people bathing naked in the canal that some would call gypsies. I also appreciated hearing my husband's stories about funny interactions during telemedicine research. Once we got to Kentucky, there were lots of stories about his interactions with the students and residents. Second only to his family, I think writing always made him happy, much like fostering medically fragile infants did for me.

## Oldest Adult Daughter

There are many things that my dad taught me directly over the years, including how to use various tools, the names and life cycles of gulf sea creatures, and the history of Savannah, but much of what I learned from him was through his example, which I can now view from the lens of my own professional life. I remember him coming home and taking time alone before we all gathered in the living room and the hushed conversations after the kids left the dinner table about a challenging patient experience or frustrations with systems and workplace dynamics. I know this now as the essential daily disconnecting and processing that sustains an academic clinician. While he did not violate patient privacy or expose us to inappropriate content when we were young, reading his recent recollections highlights the intensity of his work and the space it filled in his mind daily.

His inclination and passion for teaching also impacted our home lives, as we hosted student or resident welcome parties with table tennis in addition to receiving his guidance in finding our own ways through our training and preparation for adult life, reflecting the pipeline approach that has been a hallmark of his career. As a preteen, he and I sat in a lunch café and discussed my interests of writing and psychology, and he suggested that I could one day write about my work in addition to my hopes to produce fiction and poetry. He arranged shadow experiences where I learned about various disciplines and observed firsthand the rapport that he and others built with patients who trusted and needed them. While these experiences did not lead me to medical school (with a little help from freshman chemistry), they showed me that I did belong in relationship-building patient care. In retrospect, weekend trips to my dad's office to feed his fish, attending an evening lecture he had carefully prepared and organized in a slide carousel, and watching him interviewed as an expert on the news also prepared me for my career as a clinical psychologist in an academic medical setting.

I recall standing in his quiet office, full of books and papers and ideas, and thinking about the patients he saw in the adjacent halls and the meetings and people he saw on campus and realizing that he must be as important to them as he was to us. While I sometimes wished the time he gave others could be traded for more play in the backyard or story-telling at home, I now know that his work and home life could not be perfectly balanced. We shared our father in a way that was symbiotic and fulfilling for him, and his time and energy was for the benefit of us and countless others. The works that follow will undoubtedly paint the same picture.

**Son**

As we were growing up, my father would encourage our work in school by often saying "You know, people pay you for what you know." I saw that with his amazing opportunities outside of clinical medicine, but it was when I was able to have first-hand experience seeing his interaction with patients and co-workers that I saw why people were drawn to him. The looks of gratitude and appreciation blew me away. His essays also speak to his remarkable ability to connect on a personal level, saying what the audience needs to hear.

## Middle Adult Daughter

On Saturday mornings, my dad could be found in his study surrounded by medical journals and loose papers. He swore up and down they were very specifically distributed, and they were not to be touched. The blue rocker sat in the center, so each pile could be reached as needed. As a kid, I just knew this assortment of papers (and journals with weird pictures and big words) was important to him-but never asked why. Now that we are in the midst of our own adulthood, my dad gets to turn those papers into his dream: a collection of stories for the like-minded and the curious, with a twinkle of mystery behind the stories' truthful nature. His life's work is not just one spoke in a wheel, but many spokes working together. He has always said, "if you love your job, you will never work a day in your life". He truly found what gives him that freedom: writing.

## Younger Adult Daughter

Growing up in the household that I did, I felt special to have a father who without a doubt loved his life's work. He actually enjoyed his work so much that since I was in grade school, I went to work with him at every opportunity. When I was young it was mostly because if there was something my Daddy was doing, I felt like I should be involved, of course. I didn't really understand the importance of the space station or telemedicine, but he sure seemed happy when he talked about work. Then when in medical school myself, we were taught the importance of empathy. But it wasn't until I finally could join him in actual patient care that I understood why he loved his work so much and appreciated the real meaning of compassion and empathy.

## 4-year-old Daughter

Ready, set, go!

# TABLE OF CONTENTS

Symbolism of the Cover ....................................................................... v

Preface .................................................................................................. 1

TO MY FATHER ON HIS 89th BIRTHDAY ................................... 9

Huntsville 1983-1992 ........................................................................ 11
    Obstetrics in the Community ....................................................... 11
    Space Life Sciences ........................................................................ 28
    Clinical Stories .............................................................................. 41

University of Texas Medical Branch, Galveston 1992-1998 ............. 44
    Rural Health Support ................................................................... 44
    NASA Telemedicine instrument development ............................. 56

University of Louisville Trover Campus, Madisonville 1998- .......... 68
    Building a regional rural medical campus:
    Standing on the shoulders of giants ............................................. 68
    Obstetrics in a rural residency: Are we different? ........................ 79
    Newborn Care ............................................................................... 85
    A student directed free clinic ....................................................... 93
    Community engagement:
    Service learning as the touchstone .............................................. 108
    Getting docs to small towns: An accelerated curriculum ........... 116
    The proof is in the results: Outcomes ........................................ 124
    Developing a professional identity curriculum .......................... 134
    Developing a professional identity curriculum, Cont. ............... 145

Journal Editorial Boards:
Time to think and write, 2005-2017 ... 154

A Residency Graduation Prayer ... 188

Medical support to inpatient psychiatry unit, 2006-2021 ... 241
    Clinical stories ... 241

Covid 2020- ... 246

Discovering my own professional identity:
Finding meaning in work ... 258

APPENDIX: Original Publications ... 265

# *PREFACE*

I compiled this book not just as an act of vanity. I want to encourage others to share their stories, and if I can do it, you can too. We are all products of our upbringing. I was near retirement from a long career in clinical medicine and medical education when this came to me in a most unusual way. I had studied the career development of medical students and medical residents, resulting in a professional identity curriculum intended to facilitate their journey. I had been asked to present a summary of our model to a group of brand-new third year medical students at another medical school. They had just mastered the enormous knowledge base of the basic medical sciences and were on the precipice of immersing themselves in the care of patients. I had learned that this is a key inflection point, where some would go on to develop empathy and curiosity about the persons who came to them vulnerable and suffering, seeking help. Unfortunately, some would begin the downward slide from empathy to cynicism that comes when human suffering is reduced to organs, cells, and "the body as machine." In different ways, prominent physicians through the millennia had said that it is more important to know what person has the disease than what disease the person has.

I had done hundreds of such presentations and never really planned much in advance, as I could just speak from the heart and the sessions would go well. This time, as I looked across the sea of bright faces and began talking about how important it is to develop a physician identity, things started coming out of my mouth that surprised me. I decided to share my own journey of identity as an introduction to the concept. I was further surprised that I started my story in grade school, when my identity was "the good Catholic kid." Only later would I discover how the richness of Catholic ritual and symbolism would animate my interest in indigenous healing traditions. Next I was the smart kid, and then it became clear to me that I was a boy. The medical student smiles urged me to continue. In high school I was the really smart kid who conformed to the expectations of my all-boy, Catholic, preparatory, military school; at least while at school. Outside of school I learned from elders how to weave and throw a cast net. Only later would I learn that this was an art directly descended from the island Gullah tradition. At my first job, I worked alongside those speaking Gullah, and they shared their ancient stories with me. Then I went to a college honors program at the University of Georgia that encouraged my thirst for knowledge, which had been first initiated in high school by the Benedictine priests. In Athens I discovered my love for science and especially physiology, making my switch from ecology to pre-med an easy one. Outside of class, I for the first time had close Black friends. Walking with them on the treacherous slopes of social interactions in the 1970s, I began to understand something of their experience. Putting in the long hours studying organic chemistry, biochemistry, and animal anatomy and physiology became as comfortable as a walk on the beach. I excelled and eventually was chosen for an endowed scholarship to Vanderbilt Medical School, while all my pre-med buddies went to the state medical college. This opened unimaginable doors when I worked and studied alongside the faculty who had developed the medications that I was studying.

For these medical students, sharing my experiences during my medical school clinical years was important. Each six-to-ten-week rotation in adult medicine, pediatrics, surgery, and OB/Gyn was a thrilling ride for me, and I woke up every morning ready to learn more. Towards the end of my third year, the decision about which specialty to choose loomed large. I honestly could not imagine leaving any age group, procedure, or gender out of my future practice, and almost by chance I discovered Family Practice.

My school didn't have a department or a required FM rotation, but I stumbled onto a key mentor who opened the door for me to the joys of continuity practice. Here, every day you saw the same folks over the years, and they became far more than their diseases. A product of this same university environment, my mentor had chosen general internal medicine because that was what his role models did. But at heart he was a family doctor, and he steered me to a summer rotation in the hills of north Georgia. Two small-town family docs gave me a small place to stay on the lake, and put me on call every third night. I was terrified.

When it was my turn, I slept very little and kept lifting the receiver of the land line when it had been a while since the emergency department had called, just to be sure it still had a dial tone. I was now responsible for this group of folks in this small town, and I didn't want to let them down. Those I saw at night for minor things came back to see me in the office later and seemed genuinely appreciative. I was hooked. My enthusiasm was tested when I became aware that this village by the lake had a "Mountain Fair" where this town of about a thousand would swell to almost ten thousand for a long weekend. As I worried about this, I was occasionally called to the ED to care for those who had taken the mountain curves too fast and had significant injuries. Clearly over my head, I would begin resuscitation and basic care and ask someone to call the doc backing me up. This doc would always step into the trauma room very shortly after he was called. Only at the end of this summer experience did he reveal that he played poker late into the night with the sheriff on the nights I was on call, and they listened to the police scanner. Between that and his phone conversation with the head nurse in the ED, he would decide how quickly to come in. And he stood just outside the room, allowing me to go as far as I could safely, before stepping in. That experience was priceless.

I was relieved to hear that during the fair both docs would be on call with me, as they were for every day of the fair. Still, it was a very busy three days and I was pleased to see the sun rise on Monday morning. One case sticks in my mind. A fair reveler had a bit too much hard cider and tripped and fell down a flight of stairs, causing a fracture dislocation of his elbow. He had enough brewed analgesia on board to allow good x-rays with two views, and I knew enough about these injuries to know they could be trouble. Avoiding all the complications would be a challenge to whichever city orthopedist we chose. I was already looking in the phone book of the nearest city when the older doc walked into the ED, ordered IV antibiotics, and directed the staff to take the patient to the large procedure room in the hospital.

Knowing what would come next, I blurted out that it had only been two hours since his last Bar-B-Que sandwich, so protecting his airway was needed. With a "you worry too much" cast back over his shoulder, the older doc went to the dressing room to put on scrubs. What I saw next was amazing. The younger doc positioned himself where an anesthesiologist would and provided only mask anesthesia, with no airway protection. Just prior to going off to sleep, the patient vomited. Entirely calm, the doc removed the mask, turned him on his side, suctioned his mouth, and replaced the bag over his face. The older doc put his foot on the upper arm and as soon as the other doc said "go", he pulled hard on the lower arm. After a sickening crunch, he said "there, that should hold it. Get me the plaster." The reveler woke up and was pleased with his new wrist-to-shoulder cast.

The looks on the students' faces said that they weren't bored with old war stories yet, but I decided to abbreviate further stories so I could get to the core content of the talk. I explained that I chose UAB for my FM residency because I knew they would not limit me in maternity care training, and delivering babies was the most fun I ever had at work. And that provided the next addition to my identity. I was the first FM ever to get cesarean section privileges at University Hospital, so I was now an FM who did surgery. My timing was also fortuitous, as Dr. G. Gayle Stephens, a founding father of Family Practice, had just taken the Chair position at UAB. I learned the foundational concepts of our discipline at his elbow. During my residency in Birmingham was when my love of medical anthropology took hold, as I used the biopsychosocial model to understand the wide diversity of patients I served.

A little later, as faculty in Huntsville, I would become one of the first FMs in the country to do GI endoscopy, adding that to my identity. I also continued operative obstetrics and gynecology. Birthing many babies, including for that unique group of female NASA engineers, I became an honorary member of many young families. Also in Huntsville, the research skills I had learned along the way opened the door for me to be asked to contract with NASA to be the medical monitor for space station design. So now I was a space doc, with the opportunity to work with astronauts, my childhood heroes. And since the Soviets had many more years of experience with closed human systems, I hosted their premier scientists at our international conferences, and in my home. At one event, I stepped away from our Soviet guests to find my kids huddled around a retired NASA legend on our stairs. As the commander of the group that recovered Apollo astronauts after splash down, they were transfixed by his stories.

Later when I moved to Texas, my NASA connections led to contracts to study the performance of early telemedicine equipment at my practice in Dickinson, Texas. My family practice office was almost halfway between, and within an easy drive of the medical consultants at UTMB Galveston to the south and the NASA equipment engineers at NASA JSC in Clear Lake to the north. If something went awry with the testing, they could come in person to resolve the issue. I can proudly say that the telemedicine instrument pack used on shuttle and then space station was tested and proven in my office.

By this point the students in the audience were looking a little incredulous, wondering if I had made some of this stuff up. So I made the intended point that if you train as a generalist physician and keep your mind open, you can do almost anything. It occurred to me then that I had not only seized every opportunity that came my way, but I had cultivated that special skill of finding meaning and purpose in each. The rest of the session went as they usually do, and I got invited back, so I guess they weren't too bored. As I drove back to my hotel and passed under oak trees hung with only wisps of Spanish moss, I thought of Savannah, my home. That place with a rich abundance of moss everywhere formed me. In deep reverie about just how unique it was, I almost ran a red light. It was in that moment that I committed to write the series of books based in my hometown that would come later.

My next academic stop was as dean of a regional medical school in Kentucky. I continued delivering babies far longer than most docs, and loved every minute, even the scary moments. I served as President of the state Academy of Family Physicians, editor of its journal, and was on the editorial board of the state medical association journal. These positions required that I write regular editorials, and their inclusion in this book provides an incisive look into the important issues of the day. This academic position also gave me the time to delve deeply into medical history, an effort I had promised myself for years. After spending many hours in musty old books, I prepared a six-part conference series for our residents, students, and medical staff beginning with Hippocrates and continuing through to modern times. This gave me the matrix for the books that had been percolating in my brain for years.

The memories of complex relationships with my family and precious patients were unsettling, and for some I sought forgiveness. This wasn't easy to write about, so I did research on the early history of Savannah as a way to get started. I combined this with my study of European, West African, and American Indian healing traditions and then it all flowed out onto the page quickly.

That series of books was not comfortable for the reader who prefers linear progression. My mind moved seamlessly across time and space, as stories from my upbringing and those from memorable patients through the years are juxtaposed with the historical events that frame the magical journey, always seeking meaning. Only in retrospect did the concept of "clinical jazz" best describe my variant of stream of consciousness narrative. This concept holds that the accepted clinical guidelines, dogma that they are, are the equivalent of the written jazz score. The best physicians know when to improvise, riffing away from the score when needed to connect and heal their patient. My solidly Catholic upbringing in Savannah provided the score; everything that followed was improvisation, and each riff seemed like it belonged in the books of the *Healing Savannah* trilogy, providing a lasting record of my pursuit of meaning.

So in the first book, *Savannah's Hoodoo Doctor: The Tyranny of Dogma*, I discovered and shared the rich Hoodoo tradition among the Gullah peoples brought from West Africa, who thrived almost 300 years ago near Savannah. If you look closely enough, you can still see remnants today, and I experienced it first-hand in high school without having a name for it. In the first book I made a case that the Hoodoo concepts of healing are remarkably similar to the biopsychosocial model that I learned from Dr. Stephens. By the end of that book, I felt strangely comfortable considering myself to be a Hoodoo doctor. At the same time, I re-discovered the rich healing tradition of the indigenous Creek Indians near Savannah, and again made the case that these three healing traditions are much more alike than different. Bringing this healing comparison into the crucible of Sherman's march to Savannah and the horrors of a downtown Savannah hotel turned hospital seemed a good vehicle.

The second book, *Savannah's Bethesda: Healing for all*, is based at the Bethesda orphanage twenty years before the American Revolution, and fleshes out details of the West African healing rituals. This requires an overview of the history of slavery in America, which remarkably begins in Africa almost a thousand years before the American Civil War. The third book, set during the Siege of Savannah, does the same for the Vodou tradition brought from what would become Haiti, and weaves in the remarkable story of Count Casimir Pulaski. The third book, *Resilience Knows No Gender*, also dives deeply into gender conformation. To me these are all portions of the mosaic that has formed modern Savannah, and therefore, formed me.

Portions of this preface were used in the books of the *Healing Savannah* trilogy. The book that follows here is intended to chronicle heartfelt perspectives of interesting times in the life of that good Catholic kid from Savannah. It is in the style of the virtual reporter, where the author writes in the third person the answers to the reporter's question: "What does the reader need to understand about your experiences during the time you wrote this piece?" Those with short attention spans can start with the last two essays. I intend for the essentials of meaning in work to be found in these pages. Readers can decide for themselves.

Bill Crump, M.D

# TO MY FATHER ON HIS 89TH BIRTHDAY

*What do you say to the man who has everything?*

What can you say about the man?
He has everything

What can you say?
He taught you everything about everything

Where does wisdom come from?
I think it comes from him

Where does that twinkle live?
In his eye and in his heart

Was I a twinkle once?
I sure am glad I'm his

How does one be both firm and loving?
Do what he does

How to live so long and so well?
Care about others, and show it

How does one learn to be a Daddy?
Watch him closely

How to show him you love him?
Be like him

# *HUNTSVILLE 1983-1992*

## OBSTETRICS IN THE COMMUNITY

*As Dr. Crump moved from his residency in Birmingham to a faculty role at the University of Alabama-Huntsville campus in 1983, he brought with him the conviction that family physicians provide a special high quality obstetrical care, especially in Alabama's small towns. Within a few years, the medical liability crisis struck Alabama and those small town doctors who might only deliver 25 babies per year were suddenly expected to pay an annual insurance premium that was tenfold more than what they were paid for doing these deliveries, despite the evidence that family doctors were almost never sued. The state chapter supported his surveys showing how many of these doctors planned to stop delivering babies and the negative effect this would have. The articles below are examples, and formed the basis for active interactions with state lawmakers as they were considering legislation to lower liability premiums.*

**Crump WJ and Redmond DB.**
**A Survey of Family Physicians Providing Obstetrical Care:**
**A Preliminary Report.**
**Alabama Medicine.**
**March 1986; 39-40.**

A survey was mailed to all 528 members of the Alabama Chapter of the American Academy of Family Physicians in October 1985 concerning their current obstetrical care. Three Hundred and eighty-six questionnaires were returned in the first mailing, for an 83% return rate. Data from the second mailing and detailed demographics on the physicians included will be available soon. Because of the urgency of the problem, it was felt to be appropriate to report the preliminary data now.

Fifty-seven family physicians reported that they never delivered babies in their careers. Eighty-three still deliver babies, with 19 of those to stop within six months. Two hundred and fifty-six have stopped delivering babies since they began practice. If we restrict our study only to the 110 family physicians who stopped delivering babies within the last five years, the impact of the malpractice crisis is the largest reason. When asked what would have to happen to make them begin obstetrics again, an improvement in the malpractice problem was the most frequent response.

In summary, this 73% sample has identified only 64 physicians who will continue to deliver babies. Approximately 70% of those who have stopped in the last five years attribute this to the malpractice climate. It is estimated from this information that the number of family physicians providing obstetrical care can be increased by 46 (72%) by changes in the current malpractice situation.

The effect that these changes may have on family practice residents in training was not measured in this survey, but is another important consideration in our state's health manpower.

**Crump WJ. Status Report:**
**Family Practice Obstetrics in Alabama—More Bad News.**
**Alabama Medicine.**
**May 1988; 47-49.**

A survey in Alabama Medicine in May 1986 revealed that of Alabama Academy of Family Physicians members, only 70 intended to continue to provide obstetrical services. Of this number, 10 were full time faculty members with residency programs. Since that time, a considerable shift in state political forces has resulted in passage of tort reform legislation intended to alleviate the burden of liability premium costs associated with family practice obstetrics. As yet, no moderation in premium increase has reached the individual physician.

In the two years since the last survey, more family physicians have ceased providing obstetrical care than expected. The purpose of this study was to quantify this progress, and describe the geographic distribution of those physicians involved.

## METHODS

In October 1985 and January 1986, a survey was mailed to all 528 members of the Alabama Chapter of the American Academy of Family Physicians concerning their current obstetrical care. With an 84% return rate, this survey identified 89 family physicians who were delivering babies. A repeat survey of these 89 was conducted by the Academy in October 1987, asking only whether they continue obstetrics. Also, included in the survey were 67 family physicians who moved into Alabama after October 1985, and the 60 family practice residents who graduated from Alabama State to practice. With the exception of one residency graduate, all of those contacted responded, for a sample of 215.

## RESULTS

Of the initial group of 89, 10 were full time faculty members with residency programs. Of the 79 family physicians in practice, 7 had moved out of Alabama, and only 21 continued to provide obstetrical care. Three of the 67 family physicians moving into Alabama deliver babies, and 5 of the 60 recent residency graduates include obstetrics in their practice, giving a total of 29. Not reflected in these results are the 18 family practice faculty members who continue to deliver, including 7 in Huntsville, 5 in Mobile, 5 in Birmingham, and 1 in Tuscaloosa.

## DISCUSSION

The 1986 survey of this group of physicians identified 60 in private practice who would continue to provide obstetrical care. The majority of the physicians who had given up this part of their practice cited problems with medical liability risk or excessive premium cost as the reason. The exodus from family practice obstetrics in Alabama is continuing, with no end in sight. It would be expected, and some say advantageous, for the occasional practitioner of obstetrics (less than 10-15 deliveries per year) to stop in the current situation. It would also be expected that older physicians might stop earlier than they had planned. However, there is no one to replace them. Only 8% of the recent residency graduates saying in Alabama included obstetrics, with most of those intending to provide this service leaving the state. The future doesn't look any brighter. A recent "straw poll" at the Huntsville program showed that while they were senior medical students making their future practice plans, 72% of the current residents thought they would eventually include obstetrics. Now that they are actually involved in their residency training, only 31% still had this intention. Two-thirds of those residents in training still committed to obstetrics planned to practice outside of Alabama. The result is that productivity and influx cannot keep up with attrition, creating a serious medical manpower problem.

When liability premiums for family physicians began to skyrocket in 1985, some observers welcomed the departure of the physicians not trained in modern obstetrics. However, the process has now gone much further. A regional network of family physicians, representative of the statewide population, had reported their obstetric cases as the Alabama Perinatal Outcome Project (APOP). There have now been several reports of their care published, demonstrating high quality outcomes, sometimes with lower intervention rates than reported from teaching hospitals. At a recent national meeting, this network was recognized as a model. Most of the APOP participants have given up obstetrics, suggesting that we have "thrown out the baby with the bathwater."

Other regions have recognized the threat to quality care that the loss of family practice obstetrics presents. A model program was recently published from Beaverhead County in Montana. When the attrition process began there, a group of concerned family physicians, nurses, and hospital administrators attacked the issue head-on. The largest issue, in Montana as in Alabama, was lack of public concern. However, an initial community survey indicated that over 90% wished to maintain obstetric services in their area. A carefully planned community forum then addressed the problem as one of access to care by women in rural areas. The economic loss to the local community was also discussed. In one very small hospital, $200,000.00 was lost in direct income for obstetrics and another 45% of pediatric volume was lost when the local family physicians gave up obstetrics. They also found that every dollar spent on medical care outside the community carried four other dollars with it. These facts make the case strongly for some kind of local subsidy to lessen the impact of increasing liability premiums.

Is family practice obstetrics in Alabama worth saving? The next few years hold the answer. It is clear that there are regional clusters of active physicians who for reasons of personal commitment or local particulars continue to provide obstetrical care. A logical plan would be to support these groups by a combination of state and local funds. This would provide access to low income mothers, while allowing the physicians to continue to deliver for local insured families, keeping local funds flowing through our small hospitals. Well trained future partners must also continue to be available to these physicians. Instead of graduating 20 family practice residents each year trained in obstetrics as our state did in 1983, we may now only need 5-10 to fill spots in these regional centers. Economics will dictate whether new centers can be redeveloped and if the production of obstetric-trained family physicians will need to be increased in the future. In the same straw poll in Huntsville, nine more residents indicated that they would choose to include obstetrics in their Alabama practice if they received financial assistance with the liability premium in return for caring for indigent patients.

The overwhelming problem now is apathy. If community family practice obstetrics is important, the leadership must come from the communities themselves. The Beaverhead County program is a blueprint for success, but it requires a small nucleus of motivated people to make it work. Is anybody out there listening?

## ACKNOWLEDGMENT

The cooperation of the Alabama Chapter of the American Academy of the Family Physicians and especially Ms. Joyce Purlong is sincerely appreciated.

Crump WJ, Marquiss C, and Pierce P.
A practice-based analysis of the impact of
family physicians' cessation of obstetric care.
Alabama Medicine. 1990; 59(12): 26-30.

## INTRODUCTION

Family physicians are leaving the practice of obstetrics in large numbers, leading to what some fear may be an "extreme patient care crisis". Increasing liability risk and high premium costs are among the reasons cited by physicians who chose to give up obstetrics. National surveys of family physicians have found that less than 50% continue to deliver babies and reports from individual states describe many counties that are without obstetric care. In Alabama, the number of physicians providing obstetric care dropped from 212 to only 70 in a five year period, and current estimates are that fewer than 30 family physicians continue to deliver babies.

While this situation presents problems for many women of childbearing age, the effects are magnified among rural women and the poor. Rural patients frequently have to drive long distances to reach physicians whose patient load may be excessively high already. Many physicians prefer not to care for the medically indigent, and those with lower socioeconomic status have a higher risk of complications. In addition, Medicaid reimbursement for those patients who have this coverage has been typically very low. These access problems may lead to significant increases in maternal and neonatal morbidity and mortality. We sought to describe the effect on the process and outcome of subsequent pregnancies among women whose family physician ceased delivering babies, as well as the patients' perceived differences between the two pregnancies.

## METHODS

The Alabama Perinatal Outcome Project (APOP) was established in 1983 to document maternal and infant outcome in pregnancies managed by family physicians in small community hospitals in Alabama. The APOP is a practice network of family physicians throughout the state which provides an unselected, primary care patient population for study. Research methods, definitions, sample bias and reliability issues for the APOP have been described previously. Nine APOP physicians at four sites who had recently stopped doing obstetrics agreed to participate in this project.

One hundred thirty-four patients were eligible for inclusion in the study as they had not had a tubal ligation after their last delivery. These patients were contacted to determine if they had experienced a subsequent delivery and if they would participate in the study. Thirty-six had not had a subsequent pregnancy. No response was received from 57 women even after several attempts were made to contact them, and 10 could not be located.

The subjects were sent a consent form which explained the purpose of the study and gave permission to obtain a copy of their medical records for this last delivery. These records were used to complete a perinatal outcome form. The perinatal outcome data allows comparisons of pregnancy, labor, and delivery variables. The data set used included data in the APOP database. With this information, the two deliveries could be compared.

A questionnaire was also completed by each participating subject. The questionnaire compared the subjects' pregnancy and delivery experience while still under the care of her regular family physician to the experience she had after the family physician stopped during obstetrics. Subjects were asked specifically how far it was from their home to the hospital where they delivered for both their previous and most recent pregnancies, the distance from their home to see a doctor for prenatal visits for both pregnancies, and whether these distances caused them any difficulties. They were also asked about the size of their support network for both pregnancies. Finally, there were two open-ended questions which asked participants to describe the differences between their most recent delivery and the previous delivery, and to describe how the medical care might have been better for the last delivery.

This report will compare the process and outcome of the two pregnancies, in addition to examining the questionnaire data from survey participants which describes the differences they perceived between the two pregnancies.

## RESULTS

After three mailings, consent forms and questionnaires were obtained from 31 subjects. Five of these subjects had their first delivery after their regular family physician had stopped doing obstetrics. Data from these five subjects is not included in comparisons of perinatal outcome data, but is included in some of the questionnaire results, where appropriate. The subjects had to drive 20-35 miles farther to see their physicians for their second delivery than they did for their first. Subjects reported having 1-2 fewer friends and relatives that they could count on for assistance within 10 miles of the hospital. Nine (35%) of the women reported that the distance to the hospital caused them problems and half reported that the distance to see their physician was a problem. Most reported a less positive relationship with the physician.

Complete perinatal outcome data was available for only 19 deliveries. There were no significant differences in labor, delivery, or infant variables. More women received an epidural during their subsequent delivery. The subjects' latter deliveries occurred in larger hospitals (mean 390 beds vs 110) and in larger towns (mean population 85100 vs 8800) than for their first delivery, all attended by family physicians. For the subsequent delivery, only 26% were attended by family physicians.

## DISCUSSION

With only 31 usable questionnaires, the response rate for the study was disappointing. Locating the eligible subjects and determining which subjects had subsequent deliveries was labor intensive. Even with repeated mailings, the rate of return for the questionnaires was very low.

Overall, it is troubling that so many women responded that the increased distance they had to travel for obstetric care caused them difficulties, particularly where the doctor-patient relationship was affected. Time lost from work and increased travel expenses may add substantially to the cost of having a baby. While no neonatal mortality or morbidity was described by respondents, one woman reported that she nearly delivered in the car on the way to the hospital and another had to be transported by ambulance. Only one woman reported cutting back on prenatal visits but the increased traveling distance for prenatal care may by more of a problem than was reported by this small sample.

Because the most motivated women would be most likely to complete and return he questionnaire, these data are likely to exaggerate the actual differences between the two deliveries. Nonetheless, a clear pattern emerges. When their local family physician was delivering, the drive for prenatal care and delivery was 15-30 minutes, and the women had 2-4 people to help them with care of other children and other practical needs.

After their family physician stopped obstetrics, they had to drive 30-60 minutes, and only had 1-2 people nearby to call on for help. Considering the demands of time and energy of young parents, this could have been a minor inconvenience or a significant crisis.

In their subsequent delivery, these women traveled to cities ten times larger, delivered in hospitals with four times more beds, and were largely cared for by obstetricians. While most tolerated these changes quite well, 42% made negative comments about the subsequent delivery, and none preferred this situation. In addition to transportation and expense issues, 23% cited some alteration in the relationship with their medical caregivers. These women suggested that the increased distance resulted in fewer doctor visits and therefore less opportunity to develop a comfortable relationship with the physician. They were also anxious about the distance to be traveled in labor, and some were uncomfortable in larger hospitals.

Previous studies have shown a correlation between maternal anxiety and poor perinatal outcome. Although this sample size was too small to detect small effects, the matched design adds considerable statistical power. These patients presented in labor with lower Bishop scores in the subsequent pregnancy. This is the reverse or the usual pattern, suggesting that these women came to the hospital earlier in the labor process because of the distance involved, or their physicians admitted them earlier, or both. This longer in hospital time could increase maternal anxiety or potentially allow iatrogenic complications.

The management of labor showed some definite differences. There was a shift away from Meperidine analgesia and Pudendal anesthesia towards epidural use. While the numbers are too small in this study to determine any effects of this change, previous studies have shown correlations between epidural use and longer labors, malrotation, and assisted deliveries. There was a trend in infant outcome towards more FHR abnormality and low one minute APGARs in these subsequent deliveries, but all of the important events were too infrequent for reliable detection in this sample size.

The intent of this study was to describe the differences in process and outcome of pregnancy care in women from rural areas when their local family physician stopped delivering babies. While the response rate was disappointing, the data show some clear differences and suggest others. Larger studies are needed to answer the pressing, critical question: "Just how important is it to maintain obstetrical care by rural family physicians?"

> *During the 1980s, it became apparent that almost all studies on obstetrics were from urban university sites that included patients who were very different from those in the community, and most of the management was by faculty and residents in training and not by community practitioners. The Alabama Perinatal Outcome Project collected 180 variables on each delivery done by family physicians in 19 small towns intended to show how style of practice and outcomes differed from previous studies. Dr. Crump established and actively managed the network and published six articles in peer-reviewed journals with the results. The one below is a good example. Previous university studies had shown a cascade effect where when a physician made the decision to discontinue watchful waiting and induce labor, a series of interventions often followed, some with complications. This group of family physicians did not show this negative cascade effect.*

Crump WJ. Oxytocin and the Induction of Labor:
Use in a Network of Community Hospitals.
Family Medicine. 1989; 21: 110-113.
Copyright Society of Teachers of Family
Medicine. Used by permission.

## ABSTRACT

This study uses a matched cohort design to compare the process and outcome of patients whose labor was induced using oxytocin with those entering labor spontaneously in a network of small community hospitals. The patients with induced labor more frequently had an arrest of dilation and had infants who showed more abnormalities of fetal heart rate. There were no differences in infant APGAR scores. The previously reported increases in epidural anesthesia, episiotomy, and assisted deliveries in patients with induced labor were not found, suggesting a significantly different style of care provided by family physicians in small community hospitals.

Oxytocin use for induction of labor has become an important part of current obstetric care. Literature reports of the frequency of induction have varied from 5%-40%. Significant maternal disease has been accepted as an indication for induction for many years, and the recent adoption of an aggressive approach to the postdate pregnancy make this a frequent cause for labor induction. Truly elective intervention is advocated by some to arrange for daytime delivery, assuring a rested patient and better staff and physician planning. In addition, the recent finding that approximately 40 minutes are required to achieve steady-state plasma concentrations after changes in intravenous oxytocin has led to a much longer interval between dosage increments during induction. Some authors have reported an increase in many interventions with patients whose labor is induced, including epidural anesthesia, episiotomy, assisted delivery, and cesarean section. Some have reported more labor abnormalities and increase in fetal distress, meconium-staining, or low APGAR scores. Some studies have also demonstrated an association with neonatal hyperbilirubinemia and potential maternal risks including water intoxication and uterine rupture, rare events in modern practice.

Most of this information has been reported from selected patient populations in tertiary care centers, making it difficult to apply the findings to obstetrical care provided to unselected patients in small community hospitals. The purpose of this study was to describe oxytocin use for labor induction in such a population, with attention to the differences in process and outcome when induced labors were compared to spontaneous labors.

## METHODS

The components of the Alabama Perinatal Outcome Project (APOP) have been described previously in detail. For this study, 19 family physicians practicing in eight small hospitals, with a mean of 63 beds and 214 deliveries per year, were included. Only one of the hospitals had an obstetrician on staff, and none had a neonatologist. Each physician personally performed all necessary procedures, including cesarean sections. The mean age of the physician population was 39 years, with ten years of practice experience and an average of five deliveries per month. Seventy-nine percent were residency trained.

A common set of definitions was used for research purposes and all deliveries during 1985, 1986 and 1987 were included in this study. Completeness, reliability, and validity measures were applied to each site, and any discrepancies were resolved by retrospective chart review by a research assistant unaware of the purpose of the study. Postdate was defined as an estimated gestation at or beyond 42 weeks and labor abnormalities were defined by Friedman's criteria. Arrest of dilation was defined as a delay in first stage requiring cesarean section, and an arrest of descent required assisted delivery or cesarean section during second stage. A baseline fetal heart rate of less than 120 beats per minute was categorized as bradycardia. Any deceleration lasting longer than two minutes was considered a prolonged deceleration. Scalp pH determinations were not performed routinely by any of the participating physicians. Assisted delivery included any forceps or vacuum extraction from any station regardless of position.

There was some variation in oxytocin protocols, but all sites began at dose of 1-3mu/min by continuous infusion, and increases were also 1-3 mu/min every 10 to 30 minutes. The goal in each case was hard contractions every 2 to 3 minutes, with one site specifying 150-220 Montevideo units. Continuous electronic monitoring during active labor was routine, but use of fetal scalp electrode and intrauterine pressure catheter (IUPC) were individualized. Five percent of the patients in spontaneous labor had an IUPC placed, compared with 21% of those in induced labor. Induction was defined as oxytocin use when labor was absent, and augmentation was defined as its use after the onset of spontaneous labor. Labor was defined as the onset of regular uterine contractions. Those patients in spontaneous labor who received oxytocin only for augmentation were included in the spontaneous labor category for analysis. The population was 41% primigravida, and the patients made an average of 8.6 prenatal visits to their physicians. Of the 2,003 patients included in the sample, 163 (8.1%) were given oxytocin to induce labor. The rates for individual physicians ranged from 1.5% to 15.4%

Initial analysis revealed a significant increase in older, white patients in the group with induced labor, as well as significantly more hypertensive and postdate patients in that group. For this reason, all subsequent analysis was performed using a matched cohort design. Ninety-one of the patients with induced labor were matched with a case in the spontaneous group for age (<22, 23-27, >28), race, parity (primipara/multipara), and presence of postdate or hypertension. After matching, there was no difference in years of school completed or number of prenatal physician visits between the two groups. Statistical analysis was carried out using chi-square with one degree of freedom as a McNemar's test for dichotomous variables, and a t test was used for continuous variables.

## RESULTS

There were significant differences in labor between the two groups. There was no difference in amniotomy or protraction disorders, but a significant increase in arrest of dilation was found. The induced group had a less favorable Bishop score on admission and experienced a longer period from rupture of membranes to delivery. Analgesia/anesthesia choices showed no significant differences. There was a non-significant trend toward an increase in primary cesarean section and a decrease in assisted deliveries, with no other differences in delivery variables or postpartum complications. Infant outcome showed the labor-induced group had more FHR abnormalities, and a trend toward more meconium staining. Secondary analysis showed that the increase in FHR abnormalities included recurrent late and variable decelerations, bradycardia, tachycardia, and prolonged decelerations, but all subgroups were small with P values in the .17 to .24 range.

## DISCUSSION

This report describes oxytocin induction as used by group of family physicians providing obstetrical in small community hospitals. There are several confounders present in any study of induction. The first are those differences in the patients themselves that make the labor induced group higher risk, independent of the induction. This is a particular problem in retrospective studies, including the majority of the reports in the literature, as well as the APOP. To control for this cofounder, some authors have excluded high-risk cases and some have used a case control design. Since the intent of this study was to describe oxytocin induction in small hospitals, it was not appropriate to exclude high-risk cases, and therefore the matched cohort design was chosen. The large number of matched variables used strengthens the value of the results but necessitates smaller groups because of the difficulty of finding "perfect matches," increasing the chances of not detecting a true difference. Using the trend toward more primary cesarean sections in the labor-induced group as an example, the probability of making this type II error can be estimated. With groups this size at $P <0.05$, there is an 80% chance of detecting a 20% difference in the two groups. This degree of power is generally acceptable, and is in fact probably underestimated because of prior matching. A stratified analysis or multiple logistic regression could have further augmented the sample size available for analysis, and may by appropriate for future study of specific APOP variables.

A second confounder in studying the process variables of induction is the difference in practice styles of the individual physicians involved. In a retrospective study from McGill University in Montreal, Smith et al found that patients whose labor was induced had more epidural anesthesia, cesarean section in primiparas, and episiotomy and assisted deliver in multiparas. Although biological factors may account for these differences, these authors note, "It is possible that, once having initiated one form of active intervention (the decision to electively induce labor), the patient and the physician more readily accept the need for further intervention." If the APOP physicians used lower total dosage of oxytocin, this also might necessitate fewer interventions. However, the protocols used actually reflected the same methods as previous studies and did not follow the more recent low-dose method suggested by Seitchik et al. Although the APOP group includes all inductions, it is noteworthy that these differences in style were not seen, suggesting that the involved physicians were less susceptible to the "cascade effect" of serial interventions.

The effect of this physician style factor can be minimized by random assignment of patients to induction. There have been attempts to address this issue by prospective randomized trials. Cole, in Glasgow, Scotland, randomly assigned women with normal pregnancies with either to induction at 39-40 weeks or awaiting spontaneous labor. Labor in the "control" group, however, was induced at 41 weeks or for any new obstetric indication. He reported that the labor induced group had less frequent meconium staining and decreased postpartum bleeding, with a trend toward a lower cesarean section rate and more frequent use of epidural analgesia. There were no differences in length of labor, IV analgesia use, or one-minute APGAR scores (five minutes scores were not reported}. Martin et al reported a randomized controlled trial in normal pregnancies from Belfast, Northern Ireland. Women in the labor-induced group used more IV analgesia and had less meconium staining. APGAR scores were similar, but there was one postdate intrapartum fetal death in the control group. In this study, the labor induced group was delivered at 39 weeks, and the labor in the control group was induced at 42 weeks or "when required for medical reasons."

Sande, in Oslo, Norway, reported a similar trial more recently, including only normal pregnancies with a bishop score ≥5. The "control" group in this study also had labor induced at 42 weeks. This study reported more epidural and less pudendal anesthesia, and a trend toward an increase in cesarean section rate in the labor-induced group. They found no differences in labor duration, postpartum bleeding, or APGAR scores, but many of the groups were very small and statistics were not reported. There are two case-control studies of induction in the literature. Vierhour et al in Rotterdam, the Netherlands, included only normal pregnancies and matched for age, parity, and nationality. The labor-induced group had shorter first stage labors, less frequent meconium staining more assisted deliveries. There were no differences in birth weight, APGAR scores, or umbilical cord blood values. Yudkin et al in Oxford, England, also included uncomplicated pregnancies and matched for age, parity, and social class. They reported that the labor-induced had a higher incidence of epidural anesthesia, fetal monitoring, forceps deliveries, and cesarean section. More babies in the labor-induced group required vigorous resuscitation, including endotracheal intubation.

All of the prospective and case-control studies focused on the effect of purely elective induction in populations of normal pregnancies. The intent of this APOP study was to describe the use of induction in all patients managed in small hospitals. For appropriate comparison reports with very few exclusions must be sought. Studies that included complicated pregnancies were all retrospective. Liston and Campbell from Aberdeen, Scotland, excluded only twin deliveries, and found that the labor induced group had more meconium staining and fetal bradycardia or tachycardia, and more five-minute APGAR scores <8. Knutzen from Cape Town, South Africa, reported that the induced group had more fetal distresses (not defined further), dysfunctional labor, and cephalopelvic disproportion. Smith's study from Montreal, discussed previously, reported a series including postdate pregnancies but excluded other "maternal disorders." The labor-induced group did show increased use of epidural anesthesia, higher cesarean section rate in primiparas, and increased use of episiotomy and assisted delivery in multiparas. There was a decreased frequency of meconium staining in the labor-induced group.

The labor induced APOP group started labor with a favorable cervical exam and had rupture of membranes earlier in labor. These patients more frequently had an arrest of dilation and demonstrated FHR abnormalities. There was not a significant difference in primary cesarean sections between the two groups. However, almost all (21 of 22) the induced Cesarean sections were done for failure to progress in first stage. In the spontaneous labor group, more were done for fetal distress or other indications (breech, genital herpes). Most of the previously reported differences in process variables, such as epidural anesthesia, episiotomy, and assisted deliveries, were not found, suggesting significant style differences. The increase in FHR abnormalities found in many of the studies, including APOP, was not reflected in outcome as measured by APGAR scores. This can be explained largely by the insensitivity of the Apgar score and the lack of specificity of FHR abnormalities.

What conclusions can be drawn from these APOP data? Comparisons to previous reports must be limited because of the remarkable difference in the demographics of the population and significant study design issues. It appears that the APOP physicians, practicing in small community hospitals, were selecting an appropriate group of patients for labor induction. By choosing intervention over continued observation, they were avoiding the potential adverse outcomes associated with postdate and hypertension. The "cost" of this decision was more arrests of dilations and FHR abnormalities. Only a well-designed randomized trial can address this cost-beneficial ratio directly. What can be said with certainty is that once a decision for induction was made, the APOP physicians did not demonstrate the cascade effect of serial interventions described previously. The overall outcome obtained in the relatively unselected APOP population including complicated pregnancies, was quite favorable.

# SPACE LIFE SCIENCES

*In the late 1980s, Marshall Space Flight Center in Huntsville was assigned the task of designing the life support systems for an orbiting manned space station. Water was by far the heaviest, and therefore, most expensive to launch of the items consumed by crews. So it was obvious that water, even including waste water, would have to be recycled on board. This was a major engineering effort that had been done only on earth and only by the Soviets in Krasnoyarsk, Siberia in a secret facility. Dr. Crump tells the story that when Marshall approached the Huntsville medical school for medical help, he was the only faculty member with research experience, so the Dean dropped by one afternoon and asked him to lead the contract effort. He politely declined, as he was busy with an active advanced obstetric practice and had a wife and four small children that he enjoyed during any extra time he found. The Dean just asked him to consider it, and dropped by again in a few days and the same interchange occurred. When the Dean next dropped by, he said that he had given Dr. Crump's name to Marshall to negotiate the contract, and it was more now than just an option. Crump dove in and learned every fitting and every pipe in the station design, and learned more about microbes in water than he ever could have imagined.*

*This was a delicate time, as the Challenger explosion had just occurred, and officials at Johnson Space Center in Houston who were responsible for the humans held Marshall's team who had built the propulsion units respon-*

sible. Johnson would have to sign off on every detail of the life support system built by Marshall. Dr. Crump contracted with microbiologists, engineers, and aerospace physicians and became the medical monitor to Space Station Freedom testbed at Marshall, meeting regularly with key Johnson Center astronaut leaders. His group planned and executed missions on the KC 135 termed the "vomit comet" because it provided repeated periods of 30 seconds of zero gravity simulation during freefall, followed again by ascent. He registered himself for such a flight as the first step in astronaut training to be a mission specialist on the shuttle. It was at this point that he discovered that no company would honor life insurance claims in the event of an accident. With four small children and a wife, his dream to be an astronaut became a path not taken. The articles below are examples of the 9 articles published during this time.

It was also the period of glasnost, and former Soviet scientists for the first time were allowed visits in the U.S. As part of a conference he directed, Dr. Crump arranged for the key Siberian life support expert to speak. Remarkably, he shared all their data that had been tightly guarded for 40 years, and was accompanied by a small intense man, a young environmental scientist, and a tall, dashing interpreter. Maybe even more remarkably, these three visited Dr. Crump in his home many times and became like extended family. This image of former American military men now with NASA connections and these former Soviet arch enemies eating Alabama barbeque together in his dining room stayed with him.

Dr. Crump tells 3 stories from this time. Early in the Russians' visit, he offered them that delightful southern brew, sweetened iced tea. Like toddlers presented with something healthy, they held their glasses gamely but never brought them near their mouth. Only later would he learn that in their country only drinks that had been brought to *a boil and consumed hot or fully imbued with vodka were considered safe from contamination. The second story was when the presumed KGB handler, that small intense man, revealed that he was part of the crew that took Francis Gary Powers into custody when his U-2 spy plane was shot down over the Soviet Union. Dr. Crump broke the awkward silence by remarking that in a different time, he and his guest could have been meeting over the barrel of a gun. His guest did not smile. The last story was when Dr. Crump remarked to the interpreter how so many countries taught English to their school-aged children while the US made minimal efforts to teach foreign languages. The interpreter simply said that the US now had hegemony. His obvious sadness was broken with a slight forced smile, and awkward silence followed. Dr. Crump said he learned a new skill of keeping quiet much of the time with this group.*

*The next opportunity that found Dr. Crump was to participate on the faculty of International Space University (ISU) to teach the life support section. This truly remarkable effort brought together 120 graduate students from 50 countries in a 10-week summer session at a campus that rotates international host sites. Students choose a track (life sciences, engineering, propulsion, law), attend seminars, and work in interdisciplinary teams to produce a scientific and business plan for a specific mission. Dr. Crump tells 2 stories that highlight the impact of the non-academic benefits of getting these young people together. There were two young female Russian medical students who were very suspicious as the session began, never being more than a foot apart at any event and dressed in 1950s style. As he walked to an early morning seminar near the end of the session, Dr. Crump noticed one of them walking along with a tall Swedish male student. She wore a modern tennis skirt and both had tennis rackets strung across their backs. Glasnost, indeed.*

*The second story was of a young Chinese woman who was painfully shy at the beginning of the session. She simply couldn't come to terms with the unisex bathrooms in the ISU temporary dorm, and fairly quickly returned home. Two weeks later after some no doubt re-instruction from her authorities, she returned. At the dance party celebrating the end of the session, Dr. Crump looked up to see her crowd surfing, being propelled along by the hands of her ISU classmates. She learned more than just space law.*

*Also during this time Dr. Crump became close to those working to design an entirely closed system in the Arizona desert. The final facility was termed Biosphere 2, and the crew of 8 entirely enclosed with no resupply for 2 years were termed biospherians. Dr. Crump communicated regularly with the life scientists on that crew, including discussions of crew tensions and minor failures of some systems. He brought his family to a conference based at the support facility, and his small children learned the greeting of placing the palm of their hand to a glass pane while a crew member did the same on the inside. The planners agreed for Dr. Crump's family to be the first family in a 3 month enclosure to follow the current mission, and his children couldn't wait. Problems with oxygen cycles and food production and disagreements among the management precluded that next mission, and he often wonders what that experience would have been like.*

*The sections below are from the Space Life Sciences textbook developed for ISU. Dr. Crump served as the life support section editor and wrote two of the chapters.*

**Fundamentals of Space Life Sciences**
**Krieger Publishing Company**
**Malabar, Florida**
**1997, Used with permission**

## FOREWORD

Heinz Oser, M.D., Chief Life Scientist, European Space Agency

Data providing the basis for the health and well-being of space travelers has been collected for more than three decades. Only recently, however, have the unique environmental conditions of spaceflight, such as weightlessness and cosmic radiation, been used as tools to probe into fundamental mechanisms and processes in almost all forms of life and their dependence on and reaction to altered physical forces.

Until now results obtained from spaceflight have been published in highly specialized journals not easily accessible to the public and often difficult to trace back for references. More significantly, however, no structured background information has been complied especially for teaching purposes. Only within the framework of the International Space University has the need for up-to-date information material stimulated the creation of this book. All relevant areas in the space life sciences are covered.

We all must be grateful to the authors and to the main editor, Dr. Susanne Churchill, for their enduring patience in compiling all the chapters which are by nature of great diversity and whose only common denominator is the use of space for research into the life sciences.

This book deserves a wide use. I am convinced that is fulfills its intended goal to educate the coming generation appropriately such that it will further the life sciences research in space on a well-informed basis. I am equally eager, however, to see its entrance into routine university lecturing add a new dimension to our current thinking of all biological processes.

## PREFACE

Susanne Churchill, Ph.D., Chair, Space Life Sciences Department, ISU

As this book at last becomes a reality, I am struck with the strength and fondness of my memories of the incredible environment surrounding this book's conception at the first International Space University (ISU) summer session at MIT in 1988. For us this was the golden age of space exploration, when all things still seemed possible, and our eager and devoted faculty was the willing engine driving this new graduate university-without-walls. ISU, dedicated to supporting the peaceful development of outer space by offering a unique multidisciplinary, multinational learning experience to those whom we hoped would be the world leaders of tomorrow, was embarking on a grand experiment. Like so many before us, we dreamed of changing the world through peaceful collaboration. Who would have guessed that our hopes of joint U.S. and U.S.S.R, now Russian, missions would actually become reality or that ISU's permanent campus in Strasbourg, France, would be a *fait accompli*?

With all these obstacles at last behind us, I would like to acknowledge the very special friends and associates who have made this effort possible. My first thanks go to the chapter authors, all of whom are good friends and or/colleagues who, like myself, agreed to do this because we believed in the need to keep the next generation as enthusiastic as we had been and who continue to believe, despite the vagaries of our several space agencies, that a strong research program is the way to the future. This book could not have happened without their generous contributions of time and energy. In particular, I would like to acknowledge the role of Dr. Bill Crump, who joined the team late in the game but nonetheless in the true ISU fashion gave 110% to his tasks as section editor (Life Support Systems) and chapter author.

## Introduction to Life Support
**William J. Crump, M.D**
**Daniel Scott Janik, M.D.**

## INTRODUCTION

Life support is the provision of a sustaining environment for living organisms. As a science, it is by its very nature interdisciplinary; the most productive study is based on the best aspects of the traditions and epistemology of engineering and the life sciences. Designing and testing a complex life support system can be a most exciting opportunity to work in a relatively new field with people of diverse interests and backgrounds.

The purpose of this prologue is to provide structure for the understanding of the subsequent chapters which deal with specific aspects of life support.

## DEFINITION

The traditional components of life support are air, water, and food. Beyond these obvious requirements, experience has shown the importance of habitability and consideration of commensal organisms. Habitability refers to those human factors which make a living environment pleasant and/or desirable. A system which marvelously provides the essentials but fails to address, for example, the psychological issues of small living environments and isolation, of the provision of "creature comforts," would not win any design competition. Commensal organisms are those life forms which are required for efficient function of complex multicellular of higher species. Whether these be nitrogen-fixing bacteria around higher plant roots or human gastrointestinal tract organisms, they will share our ride in space and must be considered life support. Anyone who has experiences diarrhea after taking oral antibiotic can easily understand what can happen when important commensals are unintentionally harmed.

In addition to biological factors, life support scientists recognize certain physical factors which are historically important. These include vibration, noise, thermal and pressure requirements, ionizing and non-ionizing radiation, electromagnetic exposure and gravitational effects.

The intended recipients of the life support system will, to a certain extent, dictate design requirements. For example, if plants are included but viewed simply as functional elements to produce oxygen and food for man and not as a life support recipient, the plant system may fail and ultimately the human recipients may die. Not only must such systems address plant-produced by-products which are harmful to humans, but also human-produced contaminates harmful to plants.

A thorough understanding of life support, like any systematic study, requires knowledge of the basic operating principles of the components. Known parameters of life cycles of organisms as well as predictable patterns of exchange and turnover the key elements, e.g., carbon, nitrogen, oxygen, and hydrogen, provide the basis for life support studies. However, the real challenge is to move to the next level, to view all these cycles as interconnected and all passengers as part of the same ecological biosphere.

## TYPES OF SUPPORT

Life support systems are generally classified as physiochemical (P/C) or bio regenerative, based on primary dependency on living or nonliving subsystems and components. While this dichotomy is commonly employed, it is in actuality illusory. All life support systems by definition include a living recipient, and it is wise to view that recipient as a dynamic subsystem with a significant effect on the system. In addition, P/C systems rapidly become biological due to microbial growth and biofilm accumulation- a situation which inevitably occurs. The intimate interrelation of these factors is particular well shown by the study of filtration devices which utilize granulated activated carbon (GAC). These water purification canisters are intended to remove chemical contaminants using physiochemical operations and are widely available for home use. The finding that these devices become heavily colonized with bacteria was initially interpreted as having a negative effect on water quality. While this is certainly true if massive overgrowth occurs, it has been found that moderate bacterial growth actually increases GAC efficiency in removing certain organic contaminants. Microbial uptake of organics may also extend the effective life of such systems. Thus, what was intended to be a simple P/C system rapidly become a bio regenerative one.

Life support systems can be designed for short-term maintenance with regular provision provided from Earth or can be considered self-contained. Key concepts in this categorization are reclamation, which means that the consumable is restored to acceptable quality standards prior to reuse, and recycling, which is continued reintroduction to and reuse of reclaimed consumables by the recipients. Mixed systems are possible and common. For example, air and water (the heaviest consumable) may be recycled, while freeze dried food, with a relatively low propulsion penalty, may be provisioned from Earth and stored for months until rehydration.

"Closed" systems are generally considered necessary for spaceflight, with a truly "open" system being one which shares a planetary source of consumables. A system which is closed in matter may also receive an outside energy source, such as sunlight. In reality, closure is a continuum, and most systems vary over time with respect to their degree of closure. Closely associated with the concept of closure is that of sink size. A sink is any subsystem (or organism) which functionally removes any substance from the larger system. This can be through trapping and storing for future removal or chemical/biological transformation to a compound more acceptable to the recipients. Although the same principles apply, a system with larger sinks is more forgiving, and allows design specifications to be less precise. However, as recently discovered in the system with the largest sinks known, even the Earth has bio regenerative limits. Source and sink size are critical determinants in the design specifications of life support testbeds and systems.

A unique form of life support system is the space suit, or other forms of personal life support such as the small rail-based manned maneuvering vehicle once envisioned for space stations. These systems have very small sources and sinks; they are generally intended for individual durations of use of 3-8 hours. Except for humidity condensate management, the issues of consumable use are of less concern than thermal and airborne contaminant control.

The allure of a system which could control itself has extended from process control to "smart" systems driven by artificial intelligence algorithms. A system capable of a high degree of autonomy would greatly decrease crew time spent controlling the environment, but would be heavily dependent on an elegant sensing network. It is very difficult to match the performance of biological sensors for sensitivity, specificity, and resiliency- perhaps best demonstrated by the detection of odors. The design of reliable self-controlling life support systems is one of the major challenges for life scientists and engineers.

## AN APPLIED CLASSIFICATION

Appropriate perspective can be gained from applying the previously developed concepts to existing or planned life support systems, often described as biospheres. This term connotes a conceptual compartmentalization, implying a spherical model of interaction and closure. The components, recipients, and type of life support on Biosphere 1 (the Earth) are familiar standards of reference. All other could then be considered artificial biospheres, intended to mimic to some degree Biosphere 1.

Terrestrial biospheres providing useful perspectives include the workplace, with a known exposure period (usually 40 hrs/week in the Unites States), relatively structured semi-closed environment, and regular removal of the recipient to a system with larger sinks. The disciplines of occupational medicine and industrial hygiene, by focusing on a relatively short list of toxicants, provide us with useful approaches to other biosphere studies. The development of environmental medicine has broadened this area of concern to all habitats, including the home. The extended duration of exposure in the home (usually more than 100 hrs/week) has highlighted the importance of such issues as active and passive cigarette smoke exposure, radon levels, and other indoor air quality issues. The rigorous application of the scientific method to these problems is an important need in the 21st century. Careful study of specialized or harsh terrestrial environments, e.g., submarines, polar facilities, or undersea habitats, will also provide important information for the student of biospherics.

Extraterrestrial biospheres include spacecraft, planetary outposts, and eventually, permanent colonies. The unique combination of size, materials composition, and difficulty of resupply makes previous spacecraft missions excellent sources of data for biosphere study. This includes the short-durations flights of the U.S. Mercury, Gemini, and STS (Space Shuttle) programs, and the U.S.S.R. Vostok, Voskhod and shorter Soyuz missions, Medium duration examples include Apollo, Skylab, and some Soyuz missions; and long durations missions include some Soyuz, Mir, and the planned International Space Station.

Research and engineering testbeds provide the laboratory for the study of life support. These facilities are earth bound attempts to control as many variables as possible, allowing the variable of interest to shift and change as it would in the modeled system, while locating the testbed as close to sophisticated laboratories and the most experienced scientists as possible. Biosphere II, within its large sinks and sources, is located near Oracle, Arizona and recently completed a 2-year closure study. The Soviet closed system studies in Bios 1, 2 and 3 near Krasnoyarsk, Siberia have provided data for almost 30 years. The U.S National Aeronautics and Space Administration (NASA) has several functioning testbeds, including the Biohome at the Stennis Research Center in Mississippi, the CELSS( Controlled Ecological Life Support System) Breadboard Testbed at Kennedy Space Center in Florida, and the Plant Crop Chamber at Ames Research Center in California. For the last several years, NASA Marshall Space Flight Center (MSFC) has been assembling the ECLSS (Environmental Control and Life Support System) testbed for the space station in Huntsville, Alabama. This series of tests is the first NASA attempt to integrate multiple P/C subsystems in series to reclaim, reuse, and recycle diverse source waters including urine, hygiene effluent, and humidity condensate in a single life support system. Ground tests of P/C systems used on Mir also have been conducted in the Soviet Union. In cooperation with the University of Alabama in Huntsville (UAH), NASA MSFC has established a specialized biological plant transpiration water recovery testbed for water quality studies. Other such American industrial test beds include the Lockheed plant growth chambers in Sunnyvale, California and the Boeing plant air and transpiration water recovery chambers built and operated in collaboration with the UAH in Huntsville, Alabama. There are other testbeds, including some for military applications, some in design and others which are currently inactive.

Generally, P/C subsystems and components either work or fail. Biological subsystems and components, on the other hand, generally work in a continuously redefining environment within an envelope. As all life support systems are actually biological, the determination of the envelope for a particular system is more productive than defining its "effective life." Biological systems (such as Earth) appear more resilient than P/C systems. They have the theoretical, and in many instances functional, capacity to regenerate their biological components- often in superiorly adapted form. Failures in artificial biospheres most frequently occur from faculty sensor data. Sensing in bioprocessing systems is an area of great concern as life systems are developed.

Life support systems cause effects on recipients based on specific and combined exposures which can occur at any time. These are not necessarily static, but may change at the life support system and biological components change. These effects may confound, enhance, or mask microgravity effects and vice versa. This is of great importance for the study of gravitational biology- because perceived changes of spaceflight may actually be due to life support effects, and thus could be replicated in carefully performed ground studies. It is because of this that an understanding of life support system effects, which are by definition independent variables placed on the recipients, is absolutely necessary in order to determine the effects of the space environment on the recipients or test subjects. Detailed ground testing of the physiological effects of life support systems on recipients may in fact lead to new biomedical requirements for space, volume, contamination control, or general system performance.

The fruits of life support research for spaceflight are potentially useful on Earth. Principles learned from spacecraft with small sinks and sources provide the basis for our understanding of small, relatively closed terrestrial environments, and ultimately, spaceship Earth. The shared characteristics and value of collateral research in undersea habitats, submarines, and spacecraft, submarines, and spacecraft are obvious. However, life support concepts should also be applicable to less exotic and potentially even more important situations, such as indoor air quality. Energy efficient construction techniques in many countries have resulted in near closure of air streams in our homes. The study of concerns addressed previously of lung cancer caused by secondhand smoke or radon exposure share common concepts with life support systems. This issue has more recently grown to include increasingly closed life support systems on automobiles, trains, and airplanes, with their special exposure considerations. Life support principles will also be applicable to inhabitants of environmentally sensitive areas of Earth, where the dumping of wastes into an open system must be replaced by a more closed approach based on recycling. An especially striking application of life support science would be the design of a closed device to sustain a crew entering an area of environmental disaster (such as a nuclear accident), to allow humans to effect in situ containment quickly and safely.

A final developmental consideration of life support systems is the inherent ability of all biological systems to evolve. At some point, the compartmentalization of hardware, microbes, higher plants, animals, and man will give way to a system which takes on the characteristics of an independent organism. This process involves a fusion of animate with inanimate, where control is constantly reversed and diffused, and each component is a required part of a self-replicating system. The study of this evolutionary process is an exciting area of research for future life support scientists.

## CONCLUSIONS

The design, testing, and maintenance of life support systems to sustain living organisms is a key limiting technology for successful space habitation. Life support studies are unique multidisciplinary activities which require the most innovative approaches from the best traditions of engineering and the life sciences. The future belongs to the inquisitive.

# CLINICAL STORIES

*As his faculty medical practice grew, Dr. Crump began to enjoy recording details of a particularly touching patient story, something that would flourish later. The story below is an example.*

### MAYBE IT'S TIME.......

As we sat there in the cold silence of the ICU waiting room, myself, her husband, and my resident, my mind wandered for a moment to the first time she came into my office. A proud ex-nurse, former O.R. supervisor, she came with a well-prepared list of previous health problems and physicians with whom she had shared her care. A shattered elbow from a fall at work followed by osteomyelitis had ended her career a few years early, and abdominal pain was her only active complaint. The pain was made worse by the anti-inflammatories she took for her elbow and she wanted more H2 blockers to help balance the pain. We bargained, she agreed to some basic studies, and she left with her prescription for cimetidine in hand. I received the results of the studies: "Ultrasound positive for gallstones, upper GI positive for active duodenal ulcer," and made a plan for how our discussion would go. She didn't keep her follow-up appointment, and somehow I wasn't surprised when I received a letter from the surgeon, her former "boss," 8 weeks later: I am returning this pleasant lady to your care. Her cholecystectomy and Bilroth II gastrectomy and vagotomy went well,"

She never really recovered. I assured her that her strength would return with time, but she never ate normally again. She vomited frequently and became progressively more selective and eccentric in what she would eat.

Her husband, cared for by her in every way for most of a lifetime, began doing the shopping and buying whatever she wanted.

She wouldn't come in to see me much during her last two years. Consultations with gastroenterologists, repeat x-ray studies and endoscopies hadn't made her feel any better, and except for an occasional cimetidine, she didn't need doctors any more. When she had lost down to 89 pounds, she did come in at her husband's insistence, but he still wouldn't come in the exam room without her permission. She was vomiting many times a day now, and wouldn't listen to any discussion about depression or admission for IV therapy. She was coherent that day (competent, I thought), and left no doubt that she wanted us all to leave her alone. I bargained and dealed to no avail. I spoke with her husband separately about his coercing her into admission, but he would not violate her wishes. We agreed that when they were ready for her to go into the hospital, they would call me.

A month later, her husband called some young friends to the house. She could now not get up from the couch, and was retching almost constantly. They called us, and we saw her in the ER. Her smile was there, but the light was gone. She thought I looked familiar, and couldn't imagine what all the fuss was about. I talked with her husband, and we hoped it wasn't too late. Heroic measures: IV hydration, IV H2 blockers – maybe we could turn this thing around. It was too late. Two days later she was metabolically corrected, unable to eat and agitated and disoriented. We held on. She became incontinent, acquired a Foley, pulled her IV out twice, and 3 days later she was clearly worse.

Her husband and I talked about our options: feeding tube, hyperalimentation, let her die? We both knew in our hearts that her choice would be the last listed, but he couldn't let it happen. Here we go, I thought, down the cascade of serial interventions. Why hadn't I suggested a living will when she was coherent? We placed a nasogastric feeding tube against her resistance twice and twice she maneuvered out of the constraints and pulled it out. Our gastroenterologist tried to place a transcutaneous feeding tube, but all tissues were too friable. He suggested hyperalimentation and I acceded with a worsening sense of foreboding. She worsened further, her only response being occasional agitation.

The final episode began with a drop in blood pressure and no urinary output. The resident was called to the bedside and correctly diagnosed sepsis, urinary tract as probable source. While I was finishing with office patients, he noted no response to a fluid challenge, and considered moving her to the ICU for intensive vasopressors. Her husband, as always said "Do everything," and he did.

The silence as we sat on the soft vinyl chairs was begun by my statement that "we both know what she would want now." Maybe the plural made it easier somehow. His next words were sad and true: "Maybe it's time for us to let her go." We moved her back to her room, and vowed to do only those things that didn't seem to hurt her. The positive blood cultures, the choice of antibiotics, the discussions about an autopsy were all a blur the last few days. She would smile vacantly one day, and we would have second thoughts, but she steadily declined. She died quietly one morning with her husband at the bedside, and the smile was gone. Together we had learned to let her go.

# UNIVERSITY OF TEXAS MEDICAL BRANCH, GALVESTON 1992-1998

## RURAL HEALTH SUPPORT

*A change in the leadership of his department in Huntsville led Dr. Crump to look for an environment more supportive of his goals. There was new, innovative leadership at UTMB Family Medicine and he was one of 5 new faculty recruited to build a community-based network beyond the island. This was to include clinical training sites for the almost 800 medical students and the 30 family medicine residents who were previously confined to the island of 50,000 population. He started a practice near the bayous of Dickinson, halfway between Galveston and Houston, and welcomed 6 residents based there as well. He took an Assistant Dean role and focused on developing sites for a new integrated primary care clerkship. On his arrival there were 7 sites off the island hosting clinical medical students. When he left 6 years later, there were 750 sites across East Texas as far north as Lufkin and Nacogdoches and as far west as Victoria. He says that he went through three sets of tires on his Jeep recruiting the sites, doc to doc.*

*While speaking at a Rotary Club luncheon in the tiny town of West Columbia, he extolled the benefits of com-*

*munities hosting medical students as a way to recruit when docs retired. The problem, he said, is that finding suitable community housing for the students could be a challenge. At the end of the meeting, a tiny, frail, blue-haired lady approached him with a wary, wily expression. She had a house she could donate, but being a Texas A and M grad, she wasn't sure she could stomach giving it to the other school in Texas with that nasty longhorn steer mascot. After some lively back-and-forth, she suggested that the house be painted white and maroon and a plaque designating it as "Reveille House" positioned prominently. This was the name of the collie TAMU mascot. The deal was made.*

*As Dr. Crump travelled the backroads of the East Texas Piney woods and the sandy coastal paths west of Galveston to find community faculty, he was struck with the severity of the physician shortages, and just how stressed the existing docs were. He subsequently secured grant funding to provide practice coverage for these docs, allowing them the first break many had had in years. He himself would periodically work 60 hours over a weekend to provide this respite.*

*Dr. Crump tells a story of just how well he was treated during these shifts. He would make hospital rounds on the 3-4 patients of the local docs and then see patients in the office on Saturday morning. He carried a beeper and the staff were expected to call him day or night for emergency department patients. They put him up in a quaint old hotel downtown, and he realized when he awoke on Sunday morning that he had received no calls. After a wonderful breakfast brought to his room, he went to the hospital. There he found 2 patients waiting in the emergency department who had been there since the wee hours, and one of the hospitalized patient's pneumonia was much worse, requiring at least a change in antibiotics. When he asked the staff why he wasn't called, they politely said that they didn't usually call their docs during the night either, and they* didn't want to wake him. And, surely enough, everything necessary had been done, and there was already a verbal order waiting for his signature for the new antibiotic. As he left at the end of his shift, the staff simply said that they hoped he would be back.

One small group practice in the Piney Woods stood out. Two family docs who had completed a surgical OB fellowship succeeded in building a large OB practice and getting the OB specialist from their fellowship to join them for long periods. Dr. Crump saw this as the epitome of the style that he tried to save in Alabama, and would also periodically cover this practice and support them in any way possible. During his visits, he was provided a cabin at the nearby large lake and the use of the practice' boat.

This was the locus of another Dr. Crump story. With his wife in the front of the boat and his children in the back, he tried valiantly to deny that he was lost, but all aspects of the huge lake shoreline looked the same. It was beginning to get dark, and the tension was finally broken by the oldest leading the kids in a rousing rendition of "A three hour tour…" the theme song of the shipwrecked group on "Gilligan's Island." This was all that was needed for Dr. Crump to recognize the correct marina, dock the boat, and get everyone home before dark. One of the highlights of his frequent trips to this site in the Piney Woods was attending the local rodeo and country music performance. He and his youngest daughter had front row seats to the "Dust on the bottle" performance that would catapult a young unknown to star fame a few months later. She caught the guitar pick that he threw into the crowd as he walked off after the show. It seemed appropriate that years later his middle daughter would place that in her shoe as the "something borrowed" at her wedding. The article below is an example of innovative methods Dr. Crump developed to provide support for rural practices.

Crump, WJ, and Bersch, RB. A practice-based rural health fellowship: an innovative approach to support for rural care. Texas Medicine. November 1999; 5(11): 2-77.

## ABSTRACT

Efforts to support recruitment and retention of rural providers have sometimes included local postgraduate training. An innovative approach that included training fellows entirely in a rural area with most of the costs supported locally was found to be cost-effective and to produce the expected positive effects. Training goals and objectives were accomplished in the areas of rural health care, and the community gained an experienced provider as well as new continuing education activity. This model may be applicable to many rural sites that have adequate clinical volume, experienced and motivated local faculty, and connection to a supportive regional medical center.

## INTRODUCTION

Many methods have been tried to support rural practice. Often called recruitment and retention efforts, these methods are based on the concept that the physician is the basis of health care. Although midlevel providers play an increasingly important role in rural health, ultimately a physician must supervise and coordinate the care they provide. The successful recruitment of a physician to a small community is a powerful economic driver, with one estimate of 18 jobs generated for each physician in practice. Most recent efforts have focused on retention, with in increasing understanding that this is more difficult than recruitment, and the appreciation of the negative effects of wasted resources and failed expectations when a new physician moves on after only a short stay.

Postgraduate training in rural areas is usually conceptualized as an important method of recruitment, but providing the extra health manpower also may be an important method of decreasing isolation and providing some respite for the overworked rural physician. Rural residency tracks where the last 2 years are spent largely in a rural area have been successful but ideally are based in stable practices with at least 4 physicians. While this arrangement is preferred for residency training, by definition these communities are not among the neediest in terms of recruitment and retention.

Rural fellowship training for those who have completed a family practice residency is a more recent attempt to prepare individuals for the demands of rural practice. Often, these fellowships are focused around maternity care or other procedural training. The requirement for high clinical volume and the need to support the training program financially often dictate that much of the training time is actually spent in a metropolitan area, decreasing the experiential portion of the rural training. Our experience of a rural fellowship largely or entirely based in a rural area where providers are struggling to meet the needs of the population is presented for those considering innovations in recruiting and retaining rural providers.

## BACKGROUND

Jasper, Texas, is a town deep in the Piney Woods of East Texas, home to a population of about 10,000. The nearest secondary care is available in Beaumont, about 80 miles away, and tertiary care, in Galveston or Houston, each about 160 miles away. Before 1992, Jasper had 6 active family physicians, 1 pediatrician, and 2 small hospitals, each with a daily census of about 20. Some of the perinatal care for county residents was provided in nearby counties, with approximately 200 deliveries per year in Jasper. In 1993, the town successfully recruited 2 recent graduates of a family practice/obstetrics fellowship; they were board certified and had received advanced training in complicated and operative maternity care. Associated with increasing reimbursement for Medicaid deliveries, the practice in 1994 had built the volume to 30 to 35 deliveries per month. At this point, one of the fellowship-trained family physicians decided to leave the practice for a teaching position. This precipitated a crisis of sorts, leaving 1 family physician and 1 midlevel provider to care for this high volume mothers and babies, along with the considerable general medical population who had chosen those 2 family physicians for their care.

Working with The University of Texas Medical Branch at Galveston (UTMB), the practice provided regular rotations of senior family practice residents doing rural electives, both as a learning opportunity for the residents and as a part-time provider for the practice to meet the needs during this manpower crisis. Still, the remaining family physician had to supervise all the care given, and some months had no resident on rotation, producing an increasingly untenable situation. In the fall of 1995, the family physician was successful in soliciting the temporary assistance of an obstetrician, a former faculty member in his fellowship, to move to Jasper to assist with the maternity care. This physician came to Jasper with his long-standing interest in teaching and, especially, in fellowship development intact. Also, UTMB had successfully recruited a physician (WJC) with a long-standing interest in rural health and fellowship training. He established a formal rural health program, with practice support at the key element. The rural residency rotations were set up with Jasper and several other sites, with supplemental funding from the Texas Higher Education Coordinating Board.

With curriculum having been in place for some time and the details of a proposed budget worked out (including medical liability coverage through the university trust), recruiting fellows remained the challenge. Graduation of the next residency class was 6 months away, and the Jasper physicians were considering how many fellows they needed and could afford. The program director at UTMB was considering appropriate ways to supervise a fellow remotely, including interactive videoconferencing and telemedicine. At this point, the director was contacted by a recently graduated family physician (RBB) who, through a mutual colleague, had heard of these plans. She was interested in a short mini fellowship providing increased exposure to maternity care to facilitate the acquisition of privileges in the hospital associated with the practice she intended to join in the Northeast. A 3-month mini fellowship, based entirely in Jasper, was designed and agreed upon by both sites, including funding by the Jasper practice. At the end of the second month in Jasper, all parties indicated interest in expanding the training to a full-year fellowship experience, and this became the pilot year for the newly designed Rural Family Practice/Maternity Care Fellowship.

## Methods
### Curriculum

Based on a review of other rural fellowships, personal experience, and input from the departmental chair, goals were established. This process was important in many ways: once these goals were set, it became obvious that most if not all of them would require experiential learning, best received by living and practicing in a rural area. More specific goals this portion were established on the basis of the director's past experience in training family practice residents in maternity care. Before the decision was made to situate the training entirely in the rural area, the director of the perinatal division at UTMB approved and "signed off" on these goals, with the understanding that with so many learners in the medical center, the desired volume of procedures would be problematic. A careful documentation system, based on a perinatal outcome instrument established previously by the director, provided procedural documentation.

## SUPERVISION

Originally, the plans were for a mix of 7 to 9 months in rural area and 3 to 5 months spent in the medical center or at associated residency training sites. The time in the medical center would not allow a fellow to concentrate on very high-risk obstetrics and address other educational needs, but also would provide the director an opportunity for firsthand observation of the fellow's skills and knowledge base. This supervision at the rural site was easily established, as both the family physician and the obstetrician had extensive supervisory experience, and almost 18 months of evaluation date from the rotating residents were available to support adequate supervision. The plan for a shorter time spent in the medical center was to be facilitated by interactive videoconferencing, including the fellow as both learner and teacher in the regular residency conferences. Once funding and practical issues dictated very little time at the medical center, other methods of indirect supervision by the director were implemented.

## FUNDING

The entity providing the funding for a fellowship position must have revenue stream unless dedicated funds from another source are available.

For the existing maternity care fellowships, funding comes almost entirely from patient care revenues. Understandably, the position of the family medicine chair was that if department funds were used, the fellow would need to see the patients in departmental facilities. Although this would facilitate the maintenance of general medical skills by the fellow, continuity would be difficult, and the existing facilities already had too many learners. In addition, every day spent away from the rural site diluted the fellow's opportunities to accomplish the goals. From the perspective of those at the rural site, if they were paying the fellow's salary, they needed the fellow to see patients locally. In the end, the decision was made to fund the direct costs of the fellowship entirely from the rural site, with a mix of practice and hospital funds. The indirect costs were borne by the department as "in-kind" expenses, supplemented by both direct and in-kind support from the local Area Health Education Center (AHEC). An annualized comparison of the funding for the fellow showed 74k with that for a junior associate of 165k, if the practice were to recruit one.

## RESULTS

### Curriculum

Evaluations from the fellow and all supervisors indicated that most of the general goals were accomplished, with the exception of the goal for managed care, as this did not arise during the year. The goals for maternity care were all accomplished. The population of patients was at quite high risk. Actually, these descriptors of the patients delivering in Jasper understate the high-risk status, as some of the patients at highest risk were transferred to referral centers for delivery. However, the fellow was actively involved in the assessment, initial management, and transition to tertiary care of these patients as well. Note that most of the patients received adequate prenatal care, testimony to the access provided by these family physicians.

## SUPERVISION

On-site supervision was effective and appropriate to the level of the learner. After performing a small number of routine deliveries and being supervised by the local faculty, the fellow then acted as independent supervisor for routine deliveries done by a family practice resident. All other procedures were performed by the fellow under the direct supervision of the family physician or obstetrician on-site. As an initiative from the site, a regular weekly Grand Rounds was established. Connected by telephone conference call to the director and a specialist chosen by the fellow, controversial or difficult cases were presented and discussed. At the rural site, 8 to 15 people including nurses, nurse practitioners, and physician assistants, pharmacists, technicians, administrators, and physicians of several specialties generally attended; a category 1 continuing medical education credit was provided through a special arrangement with the AHEC. This afforded to the best opportunity for the director to supervise remotely, as the fellow's management of the cases formed the basis for most conferences, allowing for assessment and feedback from the director. These conferences were well received, suggesting that hearing the consulting specialists compliment the local care made the rural providers feel more confident in their skills. The specialists also expressed new understanding for the situation and quality of care in Jasper, and appreciated receiving the complicated cases that were necessary for training their residents and fellows in the tertiary care center.

## FUNDING

The actual salary for fellows providing maternity cate varies widely across the country, affected more by competition of recruitment than cost of living. A range of $45,000 to $120,000 was found in an informal survey by the director, so the $48,000 annual salary used in this budget was considered to be appropriate.

## OUTCOMES

The positive effects on the local community are difficult to quantify. In both written evaluations and interviews by the director, all providers indicated that the interest in improving the quality of patient care activities was augmented by having the fellow present. Her training in the Northeast brought some new perspectives to local providers. Most agreed that, rather than being perceived as a threat, her need to understand local routines of care and change them when appropriate was refreshing. Potential culture barriers were easily overcome as the fellow was received warmly by the local community, with many patients expressing their preferences to see her whenever possible. The epitome of this bonding process occurred when the fellow rode, in full western garb, in the annual rodeo parade to the cheers of the community. Perhaps the strongest measure of success was the fellow's decision to remain in Jasper as a full-time provider in the practice, serving as an active teacher in the fellowship for the subsequent year. The fellowship has grown to encompass 2 positions in Jasper, and 1 each in 2 other sites in East Texas.

## DISCUSSION

This innovative method for conducting postgraduate training entirely in a rural area was successful both from training and practice support perspectives. The approach has some similarities to the "apprenticeship" method of old. Some potential fellowship applicants have stated that if they were going to consider such an experience, they would just join an existing practice as a junior partner and not suffer the financial penalty of another year of training. The value of the experience summarized here from the fellow's perspective is that it provides another year of relatively "protected" practice for the development of skills and confidence in areas not currently provided by most residencies.

Although the focus was on maternity care, the fellow cared for 5 to 10 other inpatients daily during the year, including adult general medicine and pediatric patients, and worked in the office about 4 half-days per week. Even though her initial skills in these areas were well developed, the ability to care for these problems in a setting remote from consultants was a new experience for her. This resulted in a new "comfort zone" that ultimately led to her decision to practice in the rural area.

In a busy rural practice, a provider is often pulled among the intensive care unit, the office, and labor and delivery. A junior partner is required to respond first to what the overall practice needs her to do. However, in a fellowship setting, the learner had the freedom to choose the clinical activity that best addresses the learning objectives. In addition, the requirement of presenting difficult cases and researching the current management of each weekly, knowing that the director and consultant on the telephone will have high expectations for her, undoubtedly led to more efficient learning than would occur in typical junior associate position.

After completing this first fellowship year, the obstetrician involved moved to another practice site. Having a board-certified obstetrician-gynecologist as a local faculty for such a fellowship is probably not a requirement. However, his enthusiasm, experience, and willingness to take the extra time to teach was critical in the first year of the fellowship. In the subsequent year, the recent graduate of this fellowship and the other fellowship-trained family physician with 5 years of practice experience in Jasper largely filled this role. There was some concern that approval of observed procedures by a board-certified obstetrician-gynecologist might be important to subsequent credentialing, especially in regions where family physicians have not routinely provided advanced maternity care. To address this need and to bring more depth of experience, an obstetrician-gynecologist with almost 30 years of practice experience was added subsequently as part-time local faculty for the fellowship.

Another lesson learned was that the fellow expressed the desire, retrospectively, to have spent some time at the academic center. Her opinion was that this would have been beneficial both for educational purposes as well as for enhancing the relationship between the rural hospital and the referral center. Despite frequent urging by the director for her to do so, the bonding to the local site was so effective that she found it difficult to be unavailable to her patients and colleagues for more than just an occasional 2- to 3 day break. She had already completed the Advanced Life Support in Obstetrics provider course as a resident, so she co-taught a course with the director during her fellowship. This not only provided a refresher for her to the content of the course but allowed her to meet others providing maternity care in the region.

The positive effects on the practice and the hospital were evident, with eventual agreement to continue sharing the full cost of 2 salaries for fellows. The question arises as to whether the continued affiliation with the university is advantageous enough to justify having to work with a large bureaucracy; contracting with a university providers some challenges. From the practice's perspective, having medical liability coverage for the fellow through the university is usually an advantage. From the fellow's perspective, the oversight and sanctioning of the training by a university medical center adds considerable credibility. Although, ultimately, the list of completed procedures is the most tangible produce of the year, a letter and certificate signed by the local faculty, the director, and the department chair lend further credibility. Departmental faculty, especially the director, must feel comfortable with the level of supervision. This was accomplished by 3 to 4 site visits per year and the weekly conference calls. Technical limitations delayed the availability of interactive video with the site. When this becomes available, the director could directly observe operative procedures through a camera mounted on the operating room lights, as well as having the fellow participate more actively in medical center conferences.

Overall, the participants in this fellowship perceived a positive effect on recruiting and retaining local providers while providing a valuable postgraduate training experience. The relatively low cost of such an effort lends itself well to replication on a widespread basis. Probably hundreds of rural communities in the United States where 30 to 40 deliveries occur each month are actively seeking to recruit new providers. Where a supportive regional medical center can be connected with an interested local faculty and hospital, a special opportunity can exist to exert a positive effect on rural health care.

## ACKNOWLEDGEMENTS

This effort could not have succeeded without the support of Bud Gilliland, MD, and the vision and enthusiasm of Ed Whiting, MD. George Miller worked hard to continue the hospital support and Larry Bagby did the same for the university administration. Sam Tessen kept all the pieces balanced, and staff members of the East Texas and Piney Woods AHECs were instrumental in providing ongoing support. A small grant from the Texas Center for Rural Health initiatives augmented AHEC support for the weekly telephone conferences. Gary Hankins, MD, director of maternal-fetal medicine at UTMB, facilitated the participation of his faculty in the Grand Rounds.

# NASA TELEMEDICINE INSTRUMENT DEVELOPMENT

*While in Texas, another opportunity found Dr. Crump when one of his former NASA contacts needed a medical site to try out a compact telemedicine instrument pack to be used on Shuttle and Space Station. Dr. Crump's office in Dickinson was almost halfway between NASA-Johnson Space Center near Houston and the UTMB specialists on the island and had existing large data pipes installed. If there was a technical failure, it was a short drive for NASA contractors to repair the equipment and if the medical consultants were needed, it was a short drive to the island. The concept was to test the performance of the pack that would be used by astronauts with only brief training, directed by specialists on earth. First medical residents and then medical assistants stood in for the astronauts and the article that follows is an example of the 12 articles he would publish in what became a lifelong interest in telemedicine.*

**Crump WJ, Levy BJ and Billica RD. A Field Trial of the NASA Telemedicine Instrument Pack in a Family Practice Telemedicine Testbed. Aviation, Space, and Environmental Medicine. 1996; 67(11): 1080-1085. Used with permission.**

Background: Previous studies of telemedicine applications have demonstrated that the technology is effective but inefficient. Little attention has been directed to the primary care portion of the connection, especially the use of the medical peripheral devices. This study used a telemedicine testbed that simulates a rural practice environment to describe the effectiveness and efficiency of the NASA Telemedicine instrument Pack, a small self-contained system of medical peripheral devices. Method: This study was an 8-week field trial of a suitcase-sized pack containing a fundus camera, flexible nasopharyngoscope, dermatology macrolens, light source, and video monitor. The pack was first studied in specialty clinics and then was used in a family practice office connected to the consultant node by digital lines. Evaluations were obtained from technicians, patients, and consultants. Results: During 20 video clinics sessions, 59 patients with 38 different diagnoses were examined. The ear, nose, and throat portion of the exam was effective, with some decrement in color and clarity with compression of the signal. The eye portion was marginally effective, limited by a field of view that was too narrow and also by rigorous technician requirements. The skin exam was largely unacceptable primarily because the macrolens did not meet the requirements for color or clarity prior to compression of the signal. Conclusions: Subsequent design efforts for medical peripheral devices for telemedicine use will require significant modifications to "off the shelf" equipment to be effective and efficient. A family practice telemedicine testbed provides the appropriate environment for such field trials.

## INTRODUCTION

There has been a recent resurgence in interest in both space and Earth applications of telemedicine. NASA's interest in and use of telemedicine extends back to the beginning of human spaceflight. All of NASA's space missions have involved some degree of medical monitoring and real-time data collection on patients (astronauts) who are remote from their primary care providers (flight surgeons). In the current space shuttle program, trained crew medical officer astronauts, who may or may not be physicians, serve as physician-extenders in space for the flight surgeons back on Earth. As the space program moves into missions of longer duration, such as space station, the need to maintain crew health and performance will remain high priority to avoid costly mission effects from illness or injury, Therefore, telemedicine will play an increasingly essential role in the provision of space health care, and the need for high fidelity diagnosis and monitoring will be required to minimize unnecessary mission interruptions. The need to avoid frequent patient transport in rural health care, though of lesser magnitude per case, parallels that of space, making telemedicine applications desirable for both.

Earth applications are largely driven by cost and user acceptance, including hardware and communications aspects. For truly interactive video consultation, an image must often be obtained from a patient by way of a medical device. The perceived efficiency and user acceptance of these systems will depend heavily on the design of the medical peripherals.

Telemedicine publications in traditional medical literature have been largely descriptive, and when technologies have been critically assessed, the medical peripheral devices used are rarely described in detail. The most common description is that "off the shelf" equipment was used, meaning that a large array of separate devices, each with its own power source, is usually arrayed in an already crowded room. Although many reports cite consultant frustration, the role played by cumbersome or user unfriendly medical devices has not been addressed directly. In addition, when evaluations from the remote site have been reported, the emphasis is usually on patient acceptance of the overall technology, more focused on the images than how they were obtained. The purpose of our project was to use a testbed designed to model a rural family practice office to study the performance of a compact set of medical peripherals. The Telemedicine Instrument Park (TIP) was considered a prototype for potential applications in space as well as remote Earth applications. While designed specifically as a prototype for use in spaceflight, the advantages of small size and light weight were obviously also important for Earth applications.

## METHODS

The Telemedicine Instrument Park (TIP) resembles a small suitcase and is entirely self-contained, connecting to a standard wall outlet for power. It contains commonly used diagnostic instruments along with a small flat video monitor. The clinical assessment portion of the project was divided into two phases, each lasting approximately 4 wk. The first phase was conducted at the consultant end and functioned as a vehicle for practice and training in preparation of phase two, which involved both the consultant and primary care sites. Throughout the project, information was gathered on the TIP as a unit, the individual instruments within the TIP, the environment, specific exam procedures and clinical routines, and technical and logistical concerns. Those providing the information included specialty physician consultants, primary care physicians, clinical technicians, a process observer, and patient participants. The consultants evaluating the equipment, patient processes, and patient outcomes represented Dermatology, Ophthalmology, Otolaryngology, and Family Medicine. This project was approved in advance by the Human Use Committee of the University of Texas Medical Branch in Galveston, TX.

The first phase of the project, called the "Across the Room" phase, took place in the clinic area of the respective consultant and continued for approximately 1 month. Patient participants were selected from the existing group of patients visiting the clinic that day. The second phase of the project, the "Primary/Specialty" phase, took place where the two sites were approximately 20 mi (32km) apart. One site functioned as the model Family Practice office, with a telemedicine examination room staffed by an LVN (Licensed Vocational Nurse) and the principal investigator family physician, with the other site functioning as the consultant site, staffed by the respective consultant and project observer. For a period of 1 month, patient participants were recruited and scheduled in advance of the weekly video clinic sessions. In both phases, only non-pregnant patients 18 years of age and older were allowed to participate, all were required to give informed consent, and all were asked to complete an evaluation following the examination. During the first phase, the consultants established the sequence of the clinical exam that was used in the second phase. Information gathered throughout the project was used to develop a training plan for potential use of the TIP by NASA's flight surgeons.

Equipment evaluated throughout the project included a macro lens for examination of the skin and oropharynx; a nasopharyngoscope used for ear, nose, and throat examinations; and a fundus camera for external and internal examination of the eye. When movement of the macrolens was discovered to cause a severe decrement in clarity, such that further testing may not have been possible, a stabilizer device was attached to the lens and for the entire Primary/Specialty phase. Transmission and receipt of audio and video images was achieved from the telemedicine examination room using a tripod mounted inside the TIP. During the last session of the "Across the Room" phase and the entire "Primary/Specialty" phase, the video signal was compressed/decompressed using a Radiance (Compression Labs, Incorporated) video-conference system to facilitate transmission over a distance. During the Primary/Specialty phase, transmission was accomplished across a fiber-optic line at one-half T1 band width.

### "Across the Room" Phase

During this phase, each specialty participated weekly for 2-3 h conducting patient examinations by observing real time video images of the patient and asking questions of the patient and the technician. During the 4 wk period, 11 sessions were held, with 35 patients participating at an average exam time of 12.5 min per exam. Although the consultant was in the same room with the patient and the technician, he/she was not allowed to conduct any hands-on or "eyes-on" observation during the TIP examination.

Following each exam, the consultant completed an evaluation that captured the chief complaint, diagnosis before and after the video exam, any technical problems perceived, and answered the question, "Was a hands-on exam necessary for proper diagnosis in this case?" Each patient was given an evaluation to determine comfort and confidence level with the exam, as well as satisfaction and willingness to be examined by video in the future. Following the completion of this phase consultants were surveyed to determine the usefulness, appropriateness, and the diagnostic capability of the video examinations. The technicians who operated the equipment and facilitated the exam were also surveyed as to their comfort level and ease of use with the equipment.

### "Primary/Specialty" Phase

During this phase, participants were recruited from a family medicine practice located in Dickinson, TX. This site is approximately 20 mi from the consultant site in Galveston, TX. During a 4-wk period, patients in Dickinson were examined via video by consultants in Galveston. Each specialty held consultation sessions for approximately 2 h each week involving a total of 9 sessions and 24 patients, with an average exam time of 22 min per exam. The principal investigator and the technician (an LVN) were present at the Dickinson site and the consultants and observer were located in Galveston. Additional information was gathered on image quality, ability, and confidence regarding diagnosis, and advantages/disadvantages of the video exams.

## RESULTS

### Consultants

Consultant evaluations were collected over 2-mo period which included 20 video clinic sessions and 59 patient participants. During this time consultants from these 3 specialties saw a total of 38 different diagnoses. Although the goal of this project was to study acceptability rather than sensitivity and specificity, there was a high degree of agreement between the tentative or "working" consultant's diagnosis and the diagnosis recorded by the primary care physician during the primary/specialty phase. Of the 26 diagnoses made during this phase, only twice was there lack of concordance. In one skin diagnosis, the consultant considered squamous cell carcinoma of equal likelihood with a benign nevus, and the diagnosis on site was felt to be reliable one of the benign nevus. In the other situation, the consultants viewing the tympanic membrane felt that a perforation still existed, when examination on –site showed a fine layer of epithelium had in fact closed the perforation.

During the "Across the Room" phase, the number of times "hands-on" exam was indicated as necessary was 45 %( DERM), 20 %( ENT), and 80 %( OPH). In comparisons, the Primary/Specialty phase (across a distance) produced the following need for a "hands-on" exam: 89 %( DERM), 50 %( ENT), and 100 %( OPH). More specifically, the consultant responses were reviewed to determine how often inadequate video image served as an obstacle to making a diagnosis. While results from both phases indicated consultant concerns with the video image, the Primary/Specialty phase indicated a higher frequency of inadequate video images. In order to assess and compare the quality of audio/video output across the two phases, the consultants were asked to rate Audio, Color, and Clarity for three distinct modes using a 1 (worst) to 10 (best) scale.

Thus the Across the Room uncompressed ("Direct") can be assumed to be an assessment of the TIP subcomponents as substitutes for the consultants' eyes or usual instruments. The "Compressed Local" represents the effect of compression/decompression, and the "At a Distance" represents compression, transmission across 20 mi (32km) at one-half T1 band width, and then decompression. The decrement induced by the latter mode was noted to be different across specialty consultants. In terms of color and clarity, the ENT was fairly pleased with the instrument, and the decrement was noted to be in compression rather than distance. More specifically, detailed evaluation showed that the nasopharyngoscope performed extremely well, and the lower "direct" score was almost entirely due to the difficulty in using the macro lens for viewing the oropharynx, and the lower scores for compression were due to "tiling" from motion artifact with the macro lens and not the nasopharyngoscope. For Ophthalmology, color showed a stepwise decrement across compression and distance. Clarity was not good even when used "direct," showed no difference when compressed, and was very poor with distance. The dermatology consultants had significant problems with color and clarity during all phases. It is of note that adding the fixed light source and the stabilization device had little effect on these scores. It is also important to keep in mind that these rankings are based on a transmission rate of one-half T1, and a wider band transmission may not produce the same results.

Although not all common conditions were seen during the project, the consultants were asked to estimate, based on their experience, which common conditions could be adequately diagnosed with the TIP. Chosen from a list of common conditions in their specialty.

In considering the importance of efficiency as well as effectiveness, the time factor was measured and discussed with the consultants. During the "Across the Room" phase, average exam times for DERM and OPH were similar (8.5 mins and 9 mins, respectively) and took less than half the time of the average 20 min ENT exam. The Primary/Specialty phase, where distance was imposed, showed virtually no difference among specialties with an average exam time of 22-23 min. More subjectively, consultants were asked to compare the time required for traditional on-site clinic exams with that required to conduct a video clinic. Only one consultant indicated that each type of exam took the same amount of time. The other consultants indicated that it took considerably more time to conduct a video clinic exam.

## *Technicians*

Both technicians agreed on the importance of having a second video monitor or "picture in picture" capability allowing a view of the consultant in addition to the TIP screen which allowed only the scope or camera view. Observation and interview with the technician in the primary care setting showed that learning the technique of nasopharyngoscopy proceeded very rapidly. After observing two exams she was able in all situations to complete a satisfactory exam without "hands on" assistance. The fact that this potentially difficult exam was so easily learned provides a "calibration" for the remainder of the procedures. Thus it would be likely that this technician had far less difficulty in learning and using the equipment than an average learner would. Using the macro lens for examination of the oropharynx was exceedingly difficult. The technician could not see the patient and the screen in the same field of view, and directing the lighting and changing the focus while depressing the patient's tongue simultaneously was practically impossible. In the end, the best procedure was to focus by moving the entire camera, but it was still very difficult to depress the tongue while managing the large lens.

The technician demonstrated ease of use with the macro lens as a derm scope, once field of view and focus conventions were established. There was a tendency to zoom too close to the lesion, as most physicians are trained to view at 12-14 in focal length. The most clarity was observed by zooming all the way in first, then focusing, then moving back out to a more standard view. The stabilization device did succeed in removing one variable from the process, as the technician no longer moved the camera itself in and out from the skin.

By far the most difficult exam to master was the fundus camera. Using a standard slit-lamp head stand that was unfamiliar to the technician explained part of this difficulty. Any movement or lid droop by the patient necessitated complete reorientation of the camera. The intensity of light needed in some exams made it uncomfortable for the patient, clearly making the technician uncomfortable, feeling the need to hurry the exam. The narrow field of view provided by the camera was generally unsatisfactory to the consultant, further complicating an effective exam. Estimations from this test suggest that it would take about 5 sessions of 2 h each for an experienced LVN such as this technician to be adequately trained in the use of the fundus camera. In addition, it would be advisable for the consultant to be able to see simultaneously the technician's hand movements and the camera image to be able to guide him or her through difficult exams.

## *Patients*

The Primary/Specialty phase involved 24 participants (9 DERM, 8 ENT, and 7 OPH.) The patients generally were very positive about their exam, with 75% of the patients responding that they felt very comfortable with the exam and the remaining 25% rating it as moderately comfortable. In terms of physical comfort, only 8% (2 respondents) indicated any discomfort and both cited "bright lights" from the ophthalmology exam as the reason. Al respondents felt the consultant was "accessible," all felt their privacy and confidentiality were adequately protected, and all said that they would consider seeing a consultant by video again should the need arise.

## DISCUSSION

As the goal of the test was to discover the advantages and limitations of the TIP, it was successful. Within the constraints well-described for such field trials, important practical information about telemedicine medical peripherals was obtained. Remote examination with the TIP is perceived by consultants as requiring significantly more time than examinations in person. For Earth applications, this inefficiency is a significant obstacle to regular use. It is of note that the nasopharyngoscope, which has had much design work directed to ease-of-use, was the only application that showed no difference in duration of exam with telemedicine use. This supports the concept that design of medical peripherals is critical to the efficiency of telemedicine systems. More user-friendly equipment and a streamlined process of patient flow is also necessary to address this problem.

The macro lens as a derm scope requires some modification to be effective. The support frame was effective in decreasing motion artifact, but even less motion is desirable. The ring light appears to provide adequate light intensity, but more experience with varying degrees of diffusion is necessary to avoid the glare seen with some lesions. To address the color accuracy issue, the frame could be fitted with an opaque cover, providing an environment between the skin and the lens/camera assembly with less capacity for zoom and less adjustability of focal length might actually be preferable, as the frame will fix the focal length within a narrow margin.

The macro lens was not effective as a method to examine the oropharynx. The required instrument should have fixed focal length, a fairly wide field of view, and be easily managed with one hand. If a small lens tube with a wider field of view than the nasopharyngoscope (such as that used in some rigid endoscopes) could by adapted, this may actually be placed beyond the middle third of the tongue, removing the need for use of a tongue depressor. For this to be effective, the light tube adapter must be external to the mouth, necessitating a long lens tube to reach beyond the middle third of the tongue.

The flexible nasopharyngoscope worked quite well for visualization of the posterior nose and the posterior and inferior pharynx, as found in other reports. Although this is rarely needed either in primary care or (presumably) during spaceflight, this is an acceptable method to examine these inaccessible areas. The nasopharyngoscope as a tool to evaluate the ear is marginally effective. The inability to perform pneumatic otoscopy, so important in the diagnosis of middle ear effusions, can be partially overcome by having the patient perform a Valsalva maneuver while observing for tympanic membrane motion. This requires careful timing and a very cooperative patient, and any sound delay sometimes makes it difficult to know exactly when the patient performs the maneuver. The resolution of the tympanic membrane image is not adequate, as demonstrated by the patient with the resolving tympanic membrane perforation. To the consultant, it appeared that this perforation was till patent. Using a hand-held otoscope the onsite physician was able to discern that epithelialization across the perforation was complete, and this differentiation is important clinically. A small hand-held lens tube with a fairly wide field of view could be preferable for the ear exam. The lens tube could be fitted with a cone to function as an ear speculum. If the cone were designed to effect a tight seal, pneumatic otoscopy could be performed.

The fundus camera was significantly less effective under the constraints of this test. This instrument has functioned well in other tests, including an assessment of circulation in microgravity on space shuttle flights, and a clinical demonstration using satellite transmission. In both of these test, an extremely well trained technician and remarkably cooperative patients resulted in acceptable images. This again underscores the importance of studying prototypes in more "real world" environments prior to final design. With near perfect conditions, a narrow view of a few vessels could be obtained during the test. There is a minimal value of such a view in primary care, although an evaluation of the circulation through single vessels could be possible. Evaluating the cornea, external eye, and conjunctiva for abrasions, lacerations, and inflammation is a much higher priority need in primary care and (presumably) in space. This would be better accomplished by such a lens/camera assembly as described above, with a frame for stabilization without a head stand.

Considering these findings, the ideal instrument for a compact equipment pack would seem to be a lens tube/ camera assembly described above, perhaps fitted with a pistol grip. At one focal length (and minimal adjustability around this length), the ear, external eye, anterior nose, and oropharynx could be examined. At a second focal length, skin lesions could be optimally examined with an opaque "shroud" around the tube. For eye, nose, and skin applications, a single stabilizing bar (one each two focal lengths needed) could be threaded onto the lens tube. The distal end of the stabilizing bar (near the skin) could have a small soft pad that would rest on the skin surrounding the area to be examined (e.g., the upper maxilla for the eye). For ear exams the speculum would replace the stabilizer bar and for oropharynx exams this could be done without stabilization or by resting the bar on the upper mandible. This would greatly reduce the size and weight of the pack while increasing its effectiveness. Only miniaturization of the light source would remain as a major size/weight issue. Future tests using the established testbed will focus attention of these practical aspects of telemedicine peripheral design.

## ACKNOWLEDGMENTS

The authors would like to express their appreciation to Medical Operations at NASA Johnson Space Center, and the KRUG Life Science team who worked so hard to make this test a success, including Scott Simmons, John Pohl, and Sherry Armstrong. Oliver Black provided expert technical support and Jackie Orozco and Bebe Dwiggins managed the complex scheduling process. This project was supported by a contract with KRUG Life Sciences Medical Operations Divisions.

# UNIVERSITY OF LOUISVILLE TROVER CAMPUS, MADISONVILLE 1998-

## BUILDING A REGIONAL RURAL MEDICAL CAMPUS: STANDING ON THE SHOULDERS OF GIANTS

*The leadership changed in Galveston and Dr. Crump looked for an opportunity to use his hard-earned experience in rural health and community training of medical students while returning to "God's country." He defined this term as a state with a college football team that played in the Southeastern Conference. Another phone call out of the blue started it all. A former colleague at UTMB was now a department Chair at the University of Louisville and called to ask if he would be interested in interviewing for the dean position of a planned new regional rural medical school campus. Despite the colleague describing the need for someone with just his background, Dr. Crump politely declined. His now teenage children had just recently forgiven him for moving them from Huntsville, and they were very rooted in their gated community down the road from NASA-JSC.*

*The next time the colleague called, he made a clever proposition. He said just come and do a consultation for us as to what would be required to build such a campus. Dr. Crump bit. He tells the story that one of the first faculty leaders he met with in Louisville was the legendary Chair of the surgery department who 20 years earlier had begun sending a group of 6-8 clinical students each rotation to Madisonville for their required 8-week M-3 surgery clerkship. It had been wildly successful, and he now served on the Trover Foundation Board. Thinking he was in friendly territory, Dr. Crump described his background at the Huntsville regional campus and his rural experience in Texas, and made the case for the regional campus hosting clinical students year-round. He then made the mistake of asking the legend what he thought about that idea. The legend paused, leaned back in his chair, and simply said he thought it was the stupidest idea he had ever heard. One rotation was fine, but the other clinical experiences in small town Madisonville would clearly be inferior to that available in the big city.*

*The rest of the interviews in Louisville went fine, but Dr. Crump couldn't shake the idea that maybe Madisonville wasn't the place to put only the second US regional medical school campus that would be in a town of less than 150,000. Could this town of 20,000 in the western Kentucky coalfields provide the needed patients and faculty for all the clinical training of 24 students? It only took 3 hours in Madisonville to answer that with a solid yes. Everything about the medical center and large multispecialty clinic reminded him of Huntsville. The articles that follow detail the rich educational history of this oasis begun by the two hometown Trover boys.*

*Dr. Crump tells two stories. First, during that initial consultation, he was in the local Holiday Inn writing up his notes to make the case for a regional campus here to convince a future dean candidate, and he fell asleep. At around 2 AM, he sat bolt upright in bed, and realized this was the job for him. The second story is of his consultation exit interview with Dr. Loman Trover, the undisputed de-*

*cision maker for the enterprise. In his southern way, near the end, Dr. Trover leaned back in his chair and putting at least 3 syllables into Dr. Crump's first name, he asked "Beeall, what would it take to get you to take this job?" Dr. Crump looked around, and from Dr. Trover's glass-walled office on the eighth floor of a building taller than any other in a 60 mile radius, noted the view. He simply said that an office with a view like this would be a good start. Dr. Trover didn't smile. Dr. Crump was a bit surprised when the offer came the next day. His wife was always willing to undertake something new, but Dr. Crump says there were deep furrows all across Arkansas and Tennessee where his teenagers dug in their heels to try to stop the move.*

*The articles that follow describe the remarkable development of this award winning rural regional campus that Dr. Crump describes as built on the shoulders of giants like Dr. Trover. Almost immediately, Dr. Crump was swept up in the excitement for telehealth in Kentucky.*

## Crump WJ. Clinical Telemedicine: What is the value for the family physician? Louisville Medicine. September 2000; 48(4): 60-161.

Having practiced most of the last 20 years 30-60 minutes from my usual consultants, I have always appreciated the convenience and reassurance of the telephone consult. Once I knew the consultant well and we had shared the care of a few patients, we were each comfortable with the other's way of thinking and trusted the judgments about the intangibles of care. There were times, though, that I could tell that my specialist colleague was wondering about my ability to describe the radiograph, cardiogram, or rash in the same way he would. I am sure that there were times that my patient had to take off work or get child care, drive, find a place to park and wait to see the consultant either because the consultant was new to our system or words just could not convey what made me uncomfortable about the clinical situation.

There are many potential reasons for consultation in primary care. Some are more amenable than others to the use of electronic transmission of images or other complex data that is referred to as clinical telemedicine. To me, the key question is what added value there is to using telemedicine when compared to telephone and facsimile communication. These more conventional methods use a regular telephone line, are available almost anywhere I or my consultant happen to be, and are inexpensive. The incremental cost of a traditional telephone consult is usually about $2-3 at most for long distance charges. The basic cost of the telephone or fax machine and the telephone line is small, and can easily be justified by the many other uses for the technology. Neither I nor my consultant get paid for this consultation, but it is brief and efficient. This is the standard by which the added value of telemedicine will be measured.

My own experience with telemedicine began about 6 years ago with a telephone call from a NASA colleague I had known while I acted as medical monitor for space station design during my time of faculty practice in Huntsville, Alabama. He had heard that I had moved to Texas and started a practice in a small town about 30 minutes from Johnson Space Center. He and his group were developing a small "suitcase" of telemedicine equipment for potential use on the space shuttle and eventually on space station. They had developed a prototype, and were looking for a clinical practice site to test its capabilities.

My practice had developed into a good environment for such a study. Associated with the University of Texas Medical Branch in Galveston, we were a residency training site. Six family practice residents had their continuity practice in our office, and myself and my 3 practice associates were their faculty. As part of a departmental initiative, we had a fully electronic medical record with a computer in each exam room, connected to the full practice network of 20 other practices by digital lines. This gave us the technical support infrastructure to attempt a full motion video connection back to the campus in Galveston. Since it was a 30 minute drive one-way back to Galveston for the residents to attend required noon conferences as well as for us as faculty to attend required meetings, the idea of attending by video was very attractive. By the time my NASA colleague called, we had pretty well worked out the bugs of this connection.

This meant that a resident or faculty could finish with the last patient of the morning, walk a few feet to our small conference room to attend noon conference or faculty meeting, and then start the afternoon right on time without ever getting in their car and wasting that "windshield time." Even in the days when the video machine cost $60,000 and the digital connection was $15,000/year, it was cost effective when balanced against lost patient care time.

So we tested the equipment for NASA, having a nurse present patients from my practice to the specialists in Galveston. Remarkably, this even included fiber optic nasopharyngoscopy by the nurse, directed remotely by the consultant. Patient acceptance was very high, and the process was fairly efficient, with an average consult taking 5-10 minutes. So the clinical telemedicine we did from this site met the standard above as being almost as convenient as the telephone, and the infrastructure cost was justified by the administrative uses of the technology.

During this time we also tested various forms of store and forward equipment. This technology used regular telephone lines to establish a standard telephone call and then provided for intermittent transmission of high quality still images or short video clips during the call. These systems provided two unexpected examples of added value.

The first was while I was acting as the medical consultant to an oil rig offshore in the Gulf of Mexico. They had noticed an increasing number of skin rashes among the workers and we were going to test the resolution of the system using a cellular/radio phone to land-line connection. Since the workers rotated 2 weeks on the platform and two weeks at home and the only way to bring a worker back quickly was via helicopter (that required relatively good weather to land on the platform), the ability to keep the worker on site was a high priority. Just before the test began, one of the workers who had developed a rash became very ill and ultimately had a respiratory arrest, was intubated by the on-site nurse, and was taken via helicopter to the nearest hospital. There was now a high level of anxiety among the remaining workers, with sick-bay visits for rashes almost triple what they were previously.

Prior to the first patient visit, the nurse sent me still images of all the rashes she had archived before the incident, including the transferred patient. Then she got me access to the transferred patient's hospital records, showing that actually he had a contact dermatitis and an entirely unrelated anaphylactic reaction to a new prescription medicine he had brought on-board with him. I "examined" several of the workers on the rig who presented with rashes that were just the expected common conditions and reassured each that his situation was not like the sick worker. The result was that the planned early rotation of crews was not necessary and the number of sick calls greatly decreased. Would these men have been convinced that all was well if I had not had the capability to see their rashes? This is the issue of added value.

The second vignette occurred while we were testing the use of a short continuous data/video clip. We had a weekly Obstetrics conference with a small town 3 hours away where we had a rural fellow and a resident doing a rural rotation. They usually faxed me the fetal monitor strips that they were concerned about for our telephone discussion. Sometimes a long period of the tracing was important, and many pages had to be faxed. So, they were going to archive a large part of the tracing in advance so I could just "scroll" through it as I would have at the bedside. It just so happened that not long before we were scheduled to connect, they had a toddler present to the ED with fever and an odd rash that was developing rapidly. They captured a clip and sent it to me before we began the conference. It clearly showed that as the local examiner pressed on the rash, it did not blanch. We immediately instituted evaluation and treatment for possible meningococcemia, including targeted intravenous antibiotic treatment. Without a continuous image, I could not have discerned that the rash didn't blanch with pressure. Did this make a difference for this toddler? This is the issue of added value.

Our Commonwealth has new landmark legislation in the form of House Bill 177 sponsored by Rep. Steve Nunn. This law mandates reimbursement for telemedicine consultation and establishes a process for building a statewide communications and training network. Now as about 17 other states have done, we must begin answering the difficult question: In what situations does transmission of an image add enough value to the clinical encounter to make it worth the cost and trouble? As we proceed, the comparison to the standard of the tried-and-true telephone consult should guide our way.

**Crump WJ. The Trover Campus in Madisonville: The western Kentucky commitment to training physicians for rural areas. Journal of the Kentucky Academy of Family Physicians. November 2001; 47(4): 9-12.**

## INTRODUCTION

Almost 90% of Kentucky's counties are considered to be health profession shortage areas, having far too few primary care physicians. Despite a recent increase in the number of primary care physicians trained by U.S. medical schools, the number in non-urban areas has not changed over the last 20 years. The published literature shows clearly that doctors tend to set up practice in towns like those in which they train. The pipeline to the production of rural physicians begins with high school and continues through the retention of rural physicians in practice. This pipeline is described as "leaky," with many opportunities along the way for rural students to become attracted to big-city life during their education. This is the reason that many medical schools now have regional rural campuses that provide an opportunity for students to spend the last two years of medical school clinical training in smaller towns.

Recent studies from two traditional medical schools in Kentucky showed that there are some predictors of who will ultimately practice in rural areas in Kentucky. The study from the University of Kentucky supported the "affinity model" that suggests that a student who has a positive experience growing up in a small town is more likely to practice in similar-size town. The study from the University of Louisville also supported the affinity model, but the mathematical model was better as predicting who would not ultimately practice in a rural area.

The authors suggested that to make a significant impact, our medical schools would have to admit more of those from rural backgrounds, including some who are not currently applying. Although there are no published reports as yet, the Pikeville College School of Medicine (PCSOM) is an osteopathic initiative based on the affinity model, intended to produce physicians for rural eastern Kentucky.

## THE TROVER TRADITION IN MADISONVILLE

Education was a central element of the Trover Foundation begun almost 50 years ago in Madisonville by brothers Faull and Loman Trover. As it has developed into a modern rural integrated health system with a large multispecialty clinic and a regional tertiary care hospital, education remains in the core mission. The Trover Foundation began the first Family Practice residency in the state in 1972, and 89% of the 134 graduates practice in rural areas. Almost 28 years ago, the UL Department of Surgery began the surgery project 4-6 M-3 students at Trover each 8 week block for their required general surgery rotation.

The next phase of rural medical education at Trover began with the collaboration with UL that created the Off Campus Teaching Center (Trover Campus) in Madisonville, U of L's commitment to the regional campus concept. Begun in 1994 with a proclamation by Governor Brereton Jones, the campus had only summer programs until 1998. During 1998-2000, the campus was supported by one-time equal contributions from UL and Trover Foundation. This began the period of clinical campus activities, allowing rising third-year medical students to move from Louisville to Madisonville for their entire third and fourth years of training. During this period a permanent Associate Dean was recruited and the campus graduated 3 students, all entering FP residencies.

The summer prematriculation and preclinical programs allowed almost 60 M-1 and M-2 students to get an introduction to rural practice. At the point of the last published report, 90% of these students who had entered residencies chose primary care. In addition, since 1999 these students have completed a rural community assessment as part of their activities. These assessment reports have formed the basis for the development of health advisory councils in the four rural counties around Madisonville. In collaboration with the UK Center for Rural Health, theses advisory councils now function to guide grants for community development and further health assessments.

In 2000, despite strong endorsement from the Kentucky Academy of Family Physicians and approval by way of a formal resolution of support by the Kentucky Medical Association, the Madisonville program did not receive approval for funding from the Council on Postsecondary Education (CPE), and was continued through a special initiative from Governor Paul Patton's office using regional coal severance funds. During this time the Trover Campus further developed the pipeline activities, including college premedical programs and a High Rural Scholar program.

The high school program was developed in close collaboration and co-sponsored with the West Kentucky AHEC (WAHEC). This program placed students in health care settings in their hometowns and provided a virtual classroom to assist them with development of skills needed to increase their chances to enter and complete a premedical curriculum. Although there are other programs that give these rural students the opportunity to go to a big city for a similar experience, the negative message in these programs is that to do something really special in health care one must leave the rural area. The Trover Campus program reverses that process, bringing the classroom to the students, allowing them to discover the positive aspects of small town practice as they shadow health professionals in their hometowns. Also in 2000, an elective course in Rural Medicine for M-2 students was developed in collaboration with the KAFP. Five students enrolled the first year, and 11 are enrolled in 2001-02 year.

In 2001, the campus graduated 6 students who are now in primary care residencies (4 FP, 1 OB/Gyn and 1 Peds) and 14 are currently enrolled. A full complement of 24 students is anticipated in 2002. The High School Rural Scholar program was expanded to 20 students and the virtual classroom activities increased significantly in sophistication through collaboration with Murray State University. Students from 21 Kentucky counties have participated in the Madisonville programs so far.

## THE CURRENT CHALLENGE

The Trover campus is unique and represents the best in collaboration between an urban medical center (UL) with a commitment to train physicians who meet the state's needs and a rural integrated health system (Trover Foundation) with a 50-year experience in training students. In addition, the administrative infrastructure now includes an on-site Associate Dean, a Director of Rural Health/Student Affairs, and other support staff. This allows the further development of the necessary pipeline activities for students beyond those at U of L. Premedical students from Murray State, UK, and Kentucky Wesleyan College have participated in summer programs. Sharing of resources with the WAHEC also allows more in-depth integration of medical students from UK as well as PCSOM into the daily teaching activities occurring in and around Madisonville.

The campus does bring new costs. In addition to the personnel, the rural campus requires new funding for video-conferencing equipment, as the Trover-based students receive all the same lectures that Louisville-based students get, in real-time by interactive video connections. Fortunately, no additional facilities are required because of the contribution of existing facilities by the Trover Foundation. The challenge now is to receive full approval for continuing funding from the CPE. A proposal for Trover Campus funding was recently submitted to the CPE as the number one priority for special programs from U of L.

## THE FUTURE

Assuming that continuing funding is obtained, the Trover Campus will continue development of all aspects of the rural education pipeline. This includes active involvement with the U of L admissions process to facilitate entry of more rural students. Alost 25 years of studies show that while students from rural backgrounds (and therefore much smaller high schools) have lower overall math and science scores on the MCAT, once they are admitted to medical school, they perform on par with their urban classmates. Using the affinity model, students from small towns (whether or not they are designated Health Profession Shortage Areas) are more likely to choose small towns to practice. The Trover Campus exists to give those students another two years away from the "urban disruption" that may result in their being attracted to a big city while providing the one-to-one instruction that community-based programs offer. Activities will continue at the premedical and high school levels to prepare them for admission to medical school.

A longer rural rotation away from a tertiary care center is also planned for some Trover Campus students. The literature supports that a 4-9 month period spent training in the same rural site is highly correlated with a return to that site to practice, with the University of Minnesota's RPAP program reporting almost 30 years of success with this approach. With appropriate curriculum considerations and location of partner sites, the Trover Campus can work with individual rural sites on an RPAP model in the future.

## CONCLUSION

Based on almost 30 years of experience with regional campuses in other states, continuation of the Trover Campus is expected to place practicing physicians in Kentucky's smaller towns. This will begin to address the many health problems created by inadequate access to medical care. In addition, physician recruitment is a powerful economic engine for Kentucky's small towns. The Trover Campus rural training pipeline activities promote health careers at the high school and college applicants from small towns. This initiative is a unique collaboration, carefully crafted and proven by the first 3 years of operation, to assist development of Kentucky's rural areas into the CPE's vision of "vibrant communities offering a standard of living unsurpassed by those in other states and nations."

## ACKNOWLEDGMENTS

The continued success of the Trover Campus is based on the single-minded vision of Dr. Loman Trover, supported for almost 50 years by the leadership of the Trover Foundation. U of L has been a valued member in this collaboration, and the current strong public support of the Dean and the President is appreciated. The West Kentucky AHEC and the UK Center for Rural Health have served with us as a single seamless team to address the important health needs of western Kentucky, and we acknowledge their leadership as well.

# OBSTETRICS IN A RURAL RESIDENCY: ARE WE DIFFERENT?

*Focused on his new dean role, Dr. Crump assumed that his role delivering babies would diminish soon, but it was not to be. The family medicine residency faculty doctor designated to be the accreditation-required role model for obstetrics decided to move on. The residency director stepped into Dr. Crump's office one afternoon and asked if he'd be interested in taking on that role. Following his usual pattern, he politely declined. Rather roughly, he told the director that with plenty of obstetric providers in town already, it would require a population of pregnant patients unclaimed by anyone to provide the needed 60 continuity deliveries each year for his residents. He describes the director leaving his office looking as if his dog just died. But the next day, he returned with the thin newspaper of a small town 40 miles away with the headline "Local hospital closes delivery services." He plopped it down on Dr. Crump's desk and said that it says the 60 deliveries per year was just not enough to keep a delivering doctor in town. Wondering if it was a message from above, Dr. Crump said he would look into it.*

*For the next 20 years, he would take a resident and a medical assistant and drive to that town once per week to provide prenatal care. The women still had to go for delivery in Madisonville, but they wouldn't have to drive for their 12-15 prenatal visits with each pregnancy. When he stopped delivering babies at age 66, he had delivered well over a thousand babies from that county, including some second generation mothers. The article below shows the focus on quality of obstetric care that was a feature throughout Dr. Crump's career. It also is the first in a pattern. He created an opportunity for his young adult children to work as part-time research assistants, learn the details of research, and serve as a co-author with him. He said that this kept his enjoyment strong in what had become routine.*

Crump WJ, Wood RL, Crump SE. Continuity Maternity Care Training for Family Practice Residents: A Community Hospital Experience. Journal of the Kentucky Academy of Family Physicians. August 2003; 49(3): 10-12.

## ABSTRACT

Ensuring a good continuity experience in obstetrics is a challenge for Family Practice residency programs in small community hospitals. This report summarizes an initiative that provides for FP faculty supervision of all prenatal care and deliveries while meeting a service need in smaller communities surrounding the sponsoring hospital. Results show that the participating residents accomplished goal numbers of deliveries, including a significant increase in newborn care. Despite the slightly higher risk demographic characteristics of the FP group, good outcomes were achieved with much lower cesarean section rates. The initiative is offered as a model for those working in similar hospitals.

## INTRODUCTION

Providing a well-rounded obstetrics experience for family practice residents is a challenge for all programs, and is especially so in smaller community hospitals with a lower volume of deliveries. Although there is no minimum required for accreditation, the consensus is a guideline of 40 total deliveries with 10-15 of these from continuity patients. The process of care and multiple positive interactions over time provided by prenatal care of a continuity patient is qualitatively different from delivering a patient met first in labor. This continuity experience also allows residents to learn first-hand what the practice of obstetrics is like as they decide whether to include it in their future practice.

Until recently, many FP residency programs utilized a model where obstetricians supervised resident prenatal care and deliveries. Currently, accreditation requires each program to have one Family Physician faculty with delivery privileges, not specifying how much of the continuity prenatal care and deliveries must be supervised by this individual. The literature supports that the most successful programs have faculty who model maternity care in their own practices and exhibit competence in the delivery suite.

We report the results of an initiative designed to optimize continuity obstetrical training in a community hospital setting. Since the mid 1970s, this residency program has been known for the excellence of its graduates in adult general medicine, including inpatient care of complex patients. For the first 25 years, resident continuity patients were seen in the obstetric clinic, ideally by their primary care provider (PCP) resident, supervised by obstetricians. Deliveries were also supervised by obstetricians. In the year prior to the beginning of the initiative, residents in this 24 resident program had delivered a total of five continuity patients.

The initiative begun in 1998 included having all continuity care, including deliveries, supervised by newly hired Family Physician faculty. The central community of 20,000 population (40,000 county) was already served by five obstetricians and three certified nurse midwives, so the faculty and residents began providing prenatal care in 2 adjoining counties in affiliated clinics. At about this time, one of these county hospitals closed their delivery facility and the other county does not have a hospital. During the time period reported, the community hospital sponsoring the residency recorded 800-900 deliveries per year and had a level 2 Neonatal Intensive Care unit staffed by a neonatologist.

## METHODS

All delivery information was directly acquired from the hospital Labor and Delivery logbooks for deliveries from October 1998 to February 2003 (a 54-month period). The information gathered included deliveries performed by all obstetric providers including Family Practice Faculty, Family Practice Residents, Obstetricians and Midwives. For a 30-month period, all cases supervised by Family Practice Faculty were compared with controls consisting of 10 randomly selected deliveries per month done by other obstetric providers. Data from 300 of these comparison cases and 144 of the Family Practice deliveries were included. In addition, 22 patients were transferred from the FP service to the OB service during this time, largely because of complications or desire for elective repeat cesarean section. Because some of the prenatal care for these patients was provided by FP, these deliveries were included in the FP group for analysis. Patient information collected included: patient age, gestational age, number of prenatal visits, parity, induction, augmentation, primary or repeat cesarean section, reason for cesarean section (if applicable). Also reported were dates of delivery, time of delivery, 1 minute Apgar score, 5 minute Apgar score, choice of epidural anesthesia, and the admitting doctor for the baby. Infant admission to routine care or transfer to the Special Care Nursery was noted. All data were entered into Microsoft Excel and transferred to SPSS for further analysis.

## RESULTS

Compared to those delivered by obstetricians and midwives, the FP service had slightly more high risk demographics, including more teenage mothers and fewer multiparous patients. Despite the higher risk demographics, the patients on the FP service showed fewer preterm deliveries and a much lower cesarean section rate. The FP group showed fewer inductions, and slightly less use of labor augmentation but equal use of epidural anesthesia. The three measures of infant outcome were nearly identical in the two groups. Not included in these data are two intrauterine fetal deaths in the FP group and four in the obstetrics group. Of the newborns admitted to routine care, 86% were admitted to the FP residency service.

## DISCUSSION

The goal of providing an adequate continuity obstetric experience for these residents was accomplished while providing a needed service at the outlying clinics. Once the small hospital closed its delivery service, the patients would have had to travel 30-45 minutes one-way for each prenatal visit as well as delivery. By bringing the prenatal service to these patients, the barrier of frequent travel was removed. This would have been a significant problem, as many walked to their prenatal visits. The connection to their local hospital was important, and this was emphasized by performing all basic ultrasound studies and some laboratory tests at the local hospital, keeping this revenue local.

The patient outcome measures show that these patients benefited from FP care. The finding that, despite a slightly higher risk demographic group, FPs obtained good outcomes with lower intervention rates has been reported many times over the last 20 years. The adoption by FPs of interventions such as labor augmentation using the active management of labor strategy and judicious use of epidural anesthesia while keeping their cesarean section rate low has also been previously reported.

The initiative was not without problems, however. Scheduling residents to be out of their regular rotations for even a half-day is difficult in a community hospital that depends on the residents to cover clinical services. Each resident could not attend every prenatal session, so constant attention was required to have the patients return when their PCP was present. When this was not possible, the residents developed "buddy systems" allowing more than one resident to become familiar with each patient, a system often used in practice. The same continuity challenge was addressed at delivery when leave or other responsibilities kept the PCP from performing the delivery.

In this setting, the faculty also filled an important continuity role. During most of the time reported, only one faculty attended each clinic and delivery, so the patients came to know him well. This is efficient for the program, as FP faculty who do obstetrics are very difficult to recruit. Since the overall volume of calls is relatively low, one physician can accomplish this if time away is kept to a minimum. Each year 2-3 deliveries were staffed by the obstetric service because of absence of FP faculty. The supervision of all prenatal care by one faculty also promotes consistency and results in ongoing effective quality assurance. Each month the FP/OB faculty presented a noon conference where difficult cases or recurrent issues from the previous month were discussed.

The ultimate measure of success might be considered how many graduates include obstetrics in their subsequent practice. This is problematic because the tradition of this program was in adult general medicine, and therefore students matched to this program were pre-selected for a low level of interest in obstetrics. In addition, there are only a handful of FPs in Kentucky outside of residency programs who do obstetrics, so graduates have few practice role models or potential practice associates. More recently, the medical liability crisis has resulted in tremendous increases in premiums, making FP/OB less attractive. In the 25 years prior to this initiative, few graduates chose to include obstetrics in their practice, and none made this choice in the several years prior to the initiative. Since the initiative began, 3 have done so.

Most of the newborns reported here were admitted to the residents with faculty supervision, providing another important training opportunity. Including mostly non-pregnant adults in one's practice sharply limits the addition of new pediatric patients. Although most of these patients appropriately chose medical care for their infants closer to home after hospital discharge, the residents managed all the newborn issues. Several of the resident graduates do continue to provide newborn and infant care in their communities.

Overall this initiative provides a useful model for residency programs based in smaller communities. The future scope of the initiative will be determined by faculty stability and whether residents will be recruited who have enough interest in obstetrics to prefer more continuity deliveries.

## ACKNOWLEDGEMENT

This initiative could not have succeeded without the support of the administration and nursing staff of Regional Medical Center and the Trover Clinic. The obstetric faculty worked with us as colleagues on a single team, providing consultation as needed. Dr. Wilbon Bates participated in many of the deliveries reported, and residency support staff managed the complicated scheduling process needed to facilitate the success of the outlying prenatal clinics. Steve Fricker assisted with methodological advice and data analysis.

# NEWBORN CARE

*Periodically, Dr. Crump would be approached with opportunities to author topic-based monographs for practicing family physicians to keep them up to date and prepare them for recertification exams. The American Academy of Family Physicians was the most respected sponsor of these, and along the way he had written monographs for them on Depression and Congestive Heart Failure. Subsequently the AAFP became firmly committed to including a careful reporting of the quality of the evidence for each detail included in their monographs. Because so many practice routines had widely varying levels of quality research to support them, this easily tripled the amount of work required by the monograph authors. So, Dr. Crump usually declined these opportunities as he had enough to do building the new regional rural campus and serving as the team doctor for his daughters' soccer teams.*

*But when an Email with an opportunity to author an AAFP monograph on newborn care hit his in box, it caught his attention. It included what the practicing family doctor needed to know about screening and referral for possible autism in small children. This could provide something missing so far, an opportunity to serve as a co-author with his oldest daughter. She had completed her PhD in child psychology and was now in a leadership and clinical position with the interdisciplinary autism center in the medical center where he did his residency. He asked, and she enthusiastically accepted. What is shown below are excerpts from the product of many months of work and much back-*

*and-forth with the editors who demanded that everything had thorough documentation of the quality of the evidence.*

Crump W, O'Kelley S. Care of the Newborn. FP Essentials. Copyright American Academy of Family Physicians. August 2012; (399): 1-48. Used with permission.

## PREFACE

The family physician is in a unique position to take a family-centered approach to issues involving newborns and young infants. First-hand knowledge of the parents' traditions prior to delivery and continuing care for all members of the family provide the context for the family physician to assist families during this important and usually quite enjoyable life stage.

This edition of FP Essentials focuses on four areas of the first year of life where significant new information has been made available over the last few years. While neonatal jaundice is rarely dangerous, an elaborate system for screening and active management has become routine in many hospitals, and we review supporting evidence and the national recommendations. We will also discuss what is new about infant feeding recommendations, including some detailed management routines to facilitate successful breastfeeding. In the next section, we will review the recently updated guidelines for neonatal resuscitation, including advice for the delivering physician. Lastly, we will summarize what is known about the advantages of screening and early intervention in infants at risk for autism spectrum disorders.

We intend this issue of FP Essentials to make family physicians more comfortable with their continuing important role in caring for newborns and small infants.

## FOREWORD

Newborns should come with instructions. How many times have you heard or thought that? Even the things you learned as a physician during training sometimes seem to have missed the fine points. How yellow does this baby look? How can I best support breastfeeding in my practice or hospital? Should I use room air during newborn resuscitation? When should I consider referral of a young child with unusual behaviors? Well, short of an instruction manual, this FP Essentials may serve to fill in many of the gaps in providing care to newborns and young children.

In section one, I found the discussion of screening for hyperbilirubinemia enlightening and appreciated the review of the point-of-care tools and quick-reference treatment tables. Although breastfeeding promotion has become standard of care, section two gave me additional avenues for increasing the effectiveness of interventions supporting breastfeeding mothers and ways to quickly assess and manage common breastfeeding problems. In section three, the authors made me aware of the recent changes in the management of meconium staining and in the potential advantages, of using room air during resuscitation. Finally, the explosion of information on autism spectrum disorder has made it difficult to stay abreast of the developmental cues and optimal treatment strategies. In section four, I learned how to recognize early red flag signs and the importance of early referral for testing and management. I hope that this FP Essentials on newborn and infant care provides answers for your questions as it did for mine.

Mindy A. Smith, M.D, Associate Medical Editor

## DEFINITION OF PERVASIVE DEVELOPMENTAL DISORDERS/AUTISM SPECTRUM DISORDERS

Pervasive Developmental Disorders are a category of neurodevelopmental disorders including Autism, Asperger's Syndrome, and Pervasive Developmental Disorder Not Otherwise Specified that involve impairments in verbal and nonverbal communication, impaired social skills, and a restricted range of activities and interests. Diagnosis is based on behavioral observation and report; distinction among the three diagnostic labels depends on number of impairments observed in each symptom category and the presence or absence of language delay.

The term "Autism Spectrum Disorders" (ASD) has been used among clinicians and researchers to capture the heterogeneity of symptom presentation and functional impairment in individuals with these diagnoses. Additional evidence suggests that distinguishing the three subtypes is not reliable, even among experts in the field. Given this evolving understanding, the upcoming revision of the Diagnostic and Statistical Manual of Mental Disorders (DSM) in 2013 will subsume this set of diagnoses under a single diagnosis, ASD. The proposed revisions, however, are not without controversy among researchers, professionals, and individuals with ASD and their families.

There are at least two patterns of ASD symptom onset - an "early onset" type in which children show red flags at a very young age and follow an atypical developmental course from the beginning and a regressive type in which the child seems to develop normally in the first year of life or more and then loses previously acquired language, social, or other skills at the time that they begin to exhibit symptoms of ASD. It is unclear whether these regressive cases actually show developmental delays prior to the loss of skills. Further, current evidence supports more reliable differentiation of multiple behaviors indicative of ASD in children by age 2 years rather than in the first year of life, which makes actual onset difficult to determine.

Intellectual disability is present in between 40% and 60% of individuals with ASD. These numbers are influenced by the type of cognitive measurement (e.g., verbal vs. nonverbal measure of IQ) and the age of the individual at time of assessment (e.g., adults may show less impairment than young children, at least at the group level. Individuals with ASD exhibit a wide range of abilities and impairments, which influence response to intervention. Distinctions between "high" and "low" functioning autism are not specified in diagnostic criteria, but these terms are often used to describe the level of impairment (e.g., an individual with ASD who also has an average or above average IQ may be described as "high functioning."). The revised DSM criteria will likely allow for severity specifiers.[77] However, level of function is strongly impacted not only by an individual's obtained intellectual and adaptive skills but also the level of ASD symptom severity they exhibit.[75] Beyond the core diagnostic features, individuals with ASD often exhibit additional behavioral and emotional difficulties that impact their functioning.

## THE CASE FOR EARLY DETECTION AND INTERVENTION

Despite parental and/or professional concerns regarding development prior to age 3 years, the average age at ASD diagnosis is between 41 and

60 months .Initial caregiver concerns are usually related to language development or a noticeable loss of skills; first thoughts may include deafness. An ASD diagnosis based on comprehensive evaluation is relatively stable; the majority of children diagnosed with an ASD at age 2 years retains a diagnosis of an ASD at 9 years of age, although the specific diagnosis may change (e.g., a child with a PDD-NOS diagnosis may now meet criteria for autistic disorder). It is strongly recommended that children be referred for ASD-specific intervention, particularly those addressing communication and social development, as soon as a diagnosis of ASD is suspected, such as a child who is screened and scored in the at-risk range. A "wait and see" approach is a barrier to the early intervention that is likely to improve prognosis. We recommend that caregivers and/or providers begin with referral to the IDEA Part C lead agency for their state, as services are available for children birth through three years with disabilities, and a diagnosis of ASD is not required for eligibility.

Several experts believe that abnormalities in developing social and communication skills in toddlers with ASD can have a snowball effect where lack of basic skills (e.g., joint attention) or a heightened focus on inappropriate aspects of the environment prohibit the acquisition of more advanced and age-appropriate social skills later. For example, the child who does not develop appropriate eye gaze and social orienting is less likely to make the connection between their behavior and the reaction of others, fundamental to developing more advanced reciprocal social skills. Many current interventional approaches can potentially disrupt this chain of events and develop a new trajectory for the young child with ASD.

Children with ASD who participated in intensive early intervention services before 3 ½ years of age have been reported to have significantly better outcomes than children with ASD who did not receive services until age 5 years. Given the heritability, early detection and childhood diagnosis of ASD provides an opportunity to educate the family about the increased risk of this diagnosis among siblings and other family members. Appropriate identification of ASD can also prompt additional medical evaluation to rule out or manage contributing or comorbid factors, such as genetic conditions or seizure disorders.

## KEY PRACTICE RECOMMENDATIONS

1. **Recommendation:** Use phototherapy to reduce the risk of total bilirubin (TB) values reaching a level associated with kernicterus and the number of infants who reach a TB threshold for exchange transfusions.

   **Approved Source:** American Academy of Pediatrics (AAP)

   **Web Site:** http://aappolicy.aappublications.org/cgi/content/full/pediatrics;114/1/297.

   **Strength of evidence:** SORT B

   **Enduring material:** American Academy of Pediatrics Subcommittee on Hyperbilirubinemia. Management of hyperbilirubinemia in the newborn infant 35 or more weeks of gestation. Pediatrics. 2004;114(1):297-316.

2. **Recommendation:** Do not supplement with water or dextrose water in non-dehydrated breastfed infants to prevent hyperbilirubinemia or to decrease TB levels.

   **Approved Source:** AAP

   **Web Site:** http://aappolicy.aappublications.org/cgi/content/full/pediatrics;114/1/297.

   **Strength of evidence:** SORT B

   **Enduring material:** American Academy of Pediatrics Subcommittee on Hyperbilirubinemia. Management of hyperbilirubinemia in the newborn infant 35 or more weeks of gestation. Pediatrics. 2004;114(1):297-316.

3. **Recommendation:** Recommend and actively support breastfeeding interventions during pregnancy and after birth.

   **Approved Source:** United States Preventive Services Task Force

   **Web Site:** http://www.uspreventiveservicestaskforce.org/uspstf/usps-brfd.htm

**Strength of evidence:** SORT B

**Enduring material:** U.S. Preventive Services Task Force. Primary care interventions to promote breastfeeding: U.S. Preventive Services Task Force recommendation statement. Ann Intern Med. 2008;149(8):560-564.

4. **Recommendation:** Advise parents to begin solid foods no earlier than 4 months of age and to begin introducing solids when the infant is developmentally ready (e.g., has good head and neck control and is able to sit with support).

    **Approved Source:** AAP

    **Web Site:** http://www.healthychildren.org/English/ages-stages/baby/feeding-nutrition/pages/Switching-To-Solid-Foods.aspx.

    **Strength of evidence:** SORT B

    **Enduring material:** Committee on Nutrition of the American Academy of Pediatrics. Complementary feeding. In: Kleinman RE, ed. Pediatric Nutrition Handbook, 6th ed. Illinois: American Academy of Pediatrics, Elk Grove Village, 2009:113.

5. **Recommendation:** Use of room air could be considered for resuscitation of term newborns, given the observed mortality reduction and lack of evidence of harm; if one chooses room air as the initial gas for resuscitation, supplementary oxygen should continue to be made available.

    **Approved Source:** Cochrane Database

    **Web Site:** http://summaries.cochrane.org/CD002273/air-versus-oxygen-for-resuscitation-of-infants-at-birth.

    **Strength of evidence:** SORT B

    **Enduring material:** Tan A, Schulze A, O'Donnell CP, et al. Air versus oxygen for resuscitation of infants at birth. Cochrane Database Syst Rev. 2005 Apr 18;(2):CD002273.

6. **Recommendation:** In pregnancy complicated by meconium-stained amniotic fluid, do not use infant oral or nasopharyngeal suction on the mother's perineum or endotracheal suctioning of vigorous infants.

   **Approved Source:** AAP

   **Web Site:** http://pediatrics.aappublications.org/content/126/5/e1400.full.html.

   **Strength of evidence:** SORT B

   Enduring material: Kattwinkel J, Perlman JM, Aziz K, et al. Part 15: Neonatal resuscitation: 2010 American Heart Association Guidelines for Cardiopulmonary Resuscitation and Emergency Cardiovascular Care. Circulation 2010;122(18 Suppl 3):S909-919.

7. **Recommendation:** Incorporate surveillance and/or screening practices for developmental disabilities and autism spectrum disorder (ASD) into well-child visits. Specific screening for ASD should be conducted when parental concerns arise regarding development, particularly when concerns are related to social and communication development.

   **Strength of evidence:** SORT B

   **Enduring material:** Johnson CP, Myers SM and the Council on Children with Disabilities. Identification and evaluation of children with autism spectrum disorders. Pediatrics. 2007; 120:1183-1215.

8. **Recommendation:** Simultaneously refer for further evaluation and early intervention a child at increased risk for ASD and/or a child who shows atypical development in the areas of social and communication skills, including "red flags" for ASD, based on caregiver or professional report or observation.

   **Strength of evidence:** SORT B

   **Enduring material:** Zwaigenbaum L, Bryson S, Lord C, et al. Clinical assessment and management of toddlers with suspected autism spectrum disorder: Insights from studies of high-risk infants. Pediatrics. 2009;123(5):1383-1391.

# A STUDENT DIRECTED FREE CLINIC

*As the campus matured, a long term goal of starting a student directed free clinic materialized. Dr. Crump says that many entities in town had discussed such a project, but from his previous experience, he knew that only students could make this happen. Physicians who already occasionally wrote off the charges to uninsured patients in their offices just were not interested in volunteering their evenings to provide this care. But when wide-eyed students asked them just to precept them while they learned doctoring first hand, few could refuse. Finally a medical student with a life before medical school took this on as a cause, and it was a reality within a year. Convinced that their volunteer efforts were cost-effective and spearheaded by two summer research assistants including Dr. Crump's youngest daughter, they published the following article that was used many times in fund raising for the free clinic.*

Crump WJ, Fricker RS, Crump AM. James, T.E. Outcomes and cost savings of free clinic care. Journal of the Kentucky Medical Association. August 2006; 104(8): 340-343.

## ABSTRACT

Health care costs and client health status were measured in a 10 month period before and after an index free clinic visit for 26 poor, working, uninsured patients. A significant number of patients reported overall improvement in their health. During the period of free clinic management, the equivalent of $6500 of care was provided. Compared to utilization before the free clinic period, a savings of $33,145 was realized, largely due to decreased emergency department care and hospitalization.

# INTRODUCTION

Free clinics as a method to provide care to the uninsured are becoming increasingly important as a component of the "safety net" for these patients. The assumption is that as clients utilize free clinics, their health will improve due to easier access to care and receiving medications at little or no cost. It is also often assumed that when free clinic clients receive appropriate treatment for chronic problems and no longer have to resort to emergency department visits for outpatient care, the overall health system cost of their care will decrease.

There have been surprisingly few studies that directly address these assumptions. One of the better-designed studies in a free clinic in Rochester, Minnesota measured proxy end-points and showed a definite improvement in 72% of 109 patients. Outcomes and function were not measured, but intermediate process variables including blood pressure, HgbA1c and LDL all improved over the 100 day follow-up period. Cost was not addressed.

Another study of a free clinic in Venice, California examined the effect of pharmacists participating in the care of poor minority diabetic patients attending a free clinic and reported some improvement, limited by appointments broken by the patients. The authors compared 89 patients participating in the program with 92 diabetic patients who received services in a general clinic environment. The authors concluded that providing diabetes care to poor minority populations in a free clinic environment compares favorably to the care provided to the general population. No information was provided on cost or functional outcome. An older study acknowledged that free clinics struggle in providing optimal care due to inherent large volume demands and the variety of medical providers and volunteers found in such environments. Utilizing chart review, the authors did show modest improvements in process of contraceptive care provided to 50 women attending a free clinic in Los Angeles. Outcomes, function, and costs were not reported. A report from a free clinic serving the rural underserved in Morgantown, West Virginia provides details on the acute and chronic illnesses seen at the clinic, but provides no sample size, outcome, function, or cost data.

The focus of the study reported here is on the improvement in patient functional outcome and cost-savings of a free clinic. The Hopkins County Community Clinic was founded in April, 2004 to serve the working, uninsured poor of this mostly rural western Kentucky county. A single evening session each week is staffed primarily by medical students of the University of Louisville Trover Campus (ULTC) in Madisonville, supervised on-site by volunteer local primary care physicians. The ULTC regional Dean serves as the medical director. Paid staff includes a clinic director and, more recently, an experienced nurse. A volunteer community board sets policy for the clinic.

## METHODS

As a patient registered for their first free clinic visit (the index visit), the opportunity to join in this study was explained. A consent form and the SF-36, a functional health status form were completed by the patient. Also as part of the initial intake, the patient signed a release of information form to be sent to regional medical facilities, outpatient and inpatient, where they had received care previously.

The SF-36 survey has been validated in hundreds of studies to measure the health status of patients. It includes questions concerning physical limitations, social limitations, daily activities, pain, general mental health and resultant limitations, energy level, and perception of general health. It has been used in a variety of inpatient and outpatient settings to assess patients with cystic fibrosis, in cardiovascular and pulmonary intensive care, chronic low back pain, daily headache, and patients with known ventricular arrhythmias.

Approximately a year after the clinic began, established patients were contacted to complete another health status form and release of information form. Any patient completing both health status forms at least 6 months apart were included in this analysis. No patients were excluded on the basis of medical conditions. The charts of the 26 patients meeting the inclusion criteria were reviewed and all care received during the same period of time before and after the index visit was recorded. The care was then coded using standard CPT codes for each office visit, emergency department (ED) visit, hospital outpatient visit, and hospitalization.

Each care visit was assigned a provider cost value using Medicare RVU conversion rates effective in May, 2005. Hospitalizations were assigned the DRG payment for that condition, and ED visits were assigned a standard cost of $1000 per visit.

## RESULTS

These 26 patients had services data available for a range of 180-394 days before and after the index visit, with a mean of 284 days. As expected, these patients had a fairly high utilization of resources prior to their enrollment in the free clinic panel. This group of patients was responsible for 122 free clinic visits during the period of analysis, and 20 visits to other clinics. The free clinic physicians ordered five of the procedures, and the remainder was done as part of outside care.

The most remarkable difference was the much lower frequency of emergency department visits and hospitalizations once free clinic care was begun. Thus while the equivalent of about $6500 of care was provided in the free clinic, the cost savings was $48,240 minus $15,095, or a net of $33,145. The SF-36, as a measure of quality of life, was not expected to change greatly during this relatively brief period of study. Ten of the 11 categories of questions showed no significant difference. However, a significant number (p=.018) of these patients responded that their health was better after they began free clinic care when asked "compared to one year ago, how would you rate your health in general now?" At their first free clinic visit, 0% said their health was somewhat or much better at that time, with 36% choosing this option after their free clinic care. At their first visit, 70% said their health was somewhat or much worse, with only 39% choosing this response after their free clinic care period.

## CASE STUDIES

Two brief summaries of patients seen during the study period serve to add a human face to the numerical data.

A 22 year-old single mother, a full-time college student with no health insurance, presented to free clinic with persistent cough and fever. She had visited the ED 9 days ago for the same symptoms. The visit included lab work and a chest radiograph and she was prescribed an inhaler and an azithromycin 5- day pack. During the initial interview, she began crying, explaining that now she had a bill for almost $800. When she went to the pharmacy, she could afford the generic inhaler, but not the antibiotics. She had been unable to return to class, and a friend has had to help take care of her daughter. On examination, she had a temperature of 103.2 F, HR of 112, and RR 28. She was coughing frequently and had rales localized to the left lower posterior chest. She was diagnosed with pneumonia and given samples of an extended-spectrum erythromycin and advised to continue with the inhaler if it helped with the cough. She was seen back in a week, saying that 2 days after her free clinic visit she was able to return to class and her cough was almost gone now.

A 60 year-old woman presented to the free clinic saying that she was out of some of her heart medicines. She worked at a convenience store but had no insurance. She reported having a heart attack about a month ago, having coronary angioplasty and stent placement at that admission. She was supposed to be on 9 medicines, including a very expensive antiplatelet agent. In the initial interview, she expressed great concern that she may not be able to pay all the bills she was accumulating. She had gotten a few samples from her cardiologist and borrowed money to cover some, but had not had the more expensive ones, including the beta blocker, for about 2 weeks. She also had decided not to get the statin prescription filled because of its cost. She was now using about 2 TNG per day for her remaining angina and could not work. She received samples of most of her medicines during this first visit, and was enrolled in the patient assistance programs for all 9. Over the next six months she was able to decrease her TNG use to about twice per week, and worked 4-6 hours per day, preferring not to incur the cost of a cardiologist visit. She developed mild CHF that again caused her to stop work until her symptoms resolved with addition of an ACE Inhibitor to her regimen. About 6 months after her initial free clinic presentation she began to have frequent atypical chest pain, was admitted, and catheterization showed no significant change. The pain was felt to be GI in origin, with recommendation for proton pump inhibitor treatment. This was also provided through a patient assistance program, and her chest pain returned to the stable pattern.

## DISCUSSION

These preliminary data support the often-held belief that the working, uninsured, poor are high utilizers of health resources and that free clinic care can decrease this cost. The data, although from a very brief time, also show that the patients' quality of life was improved by free clinic care. There are several limitations inherent in this study. Despite multiple attempts to obtain records from all outside care, it is possible that not all utilization was captured. If this is true, this error should have occurred both before and after free clinic care, "canceling out" any error. In a sample this small, it is also possible that a few patients with high utilization could obscure the real pattern. Although one patient was responsible for 2 of the cardiac catheterizations (one before and one after free clinic enrollment), the real difference in cost was driven by hospital admissions and emergency department visits. These were distributed widely across the sample.

Another limitation is that in patients with chronic disease, the SF-36 may change very slowly. During the average 9.5 months of this study, it is remarkable that the most global item changed for the better. It is possible that with longer follow-up, some of the items may actually get worse. For example, access to prescription medications should increase health status. But if enough patients had negative side effects, their new access to these medicines might actually worsen health status.

These patients and the other 180 patients seen in the free clinic in the first year of operation are now participating in a registry that will allow longitudinal studies over longer periods of time with more data points. Subsequent studies may address the limitations and extend the possible conclusions.

## ACKNOWLEDGEMENTS

We express our sincere appreciation for the cooperation of our patients, the support of the free clinic board, and the hard work of all the clinic volunteers and paid staff. The Trover Foundation provided uncompensated lab tests, imaging, and some consultation for these patients. Many pharmaceutical companies provided the free medications from their assistance programs for the needy, and the University of Louisville Trover Campus provided support for data collection and analysis. A special thanks goes to Jennifer Nelson, R.N., who supervised all chart review and data collection.

*Next came time to evaluate all aspects of the free clinic. A team led by a motivated medical student and including Dr. Crump's son, who worked as a summer research assistant, published the following article.*

**Crump WJ Jr, King MA, Matera EL, Crump WJ III. Experience with a medical student-directed free clinic: Patient, student, staff, and faculty perspectives. Journal of the Kentucky Medical Association. 2011; 109: 9-14.**

## ABSTRACT

A survey of 108 patient visits to a medical student-directed free clinic in rural Western Kentucky over a 4 month period showed general satisfaction with the care provided, with a small minority suggesting improvement in time taken to get an appointment, waiting room time, and delay in receiving medication refills. Student directors have implemented specific process improvements to address these issues. The perspectives of students, staff, and faculty concerning the operation of such a clinic are also summarized for those interested in starting such an effort and future studies are suggested.

## INTRODUCTION

The benefits of student-directed free clinics for both patients and students seem evident. For patients who are uninsured, free clinics provide part of the safety net that gives them the care for chronic conditions or acute illness they often cannot get elsewhere. For medical students, the chance to practice the full range of patient care, from patient presentation to documentation, is often unparalleled by other rotations. Our 6-year experience with a student-run clinic in Hopkins County bears out these benefits. Kentucky currently has 24 free clinics. We wanted to take a closer look at perceptions of those involved with this service learning model, and offer these perspectives for those considering establishing such a free clinic.

In a comprehensive and systematic study of free clinics, Darnell found that they provide a broad range of services to 1.8 million individuals, a substantial portion of the underserved compared to the 6 million patients served by federally funded health centers. Though free clinics continue to make up a substantial part of the healthcare safety net, Darnell notes that they still operate largely outside of the formal system. Only in recent years have researchers begun to study the quality of care delivered by these providers. One such study was reported previously from the Hopkins County Community Clinic (HCCC) in Madisonville, Kentucky, a student-run clinic affiliated with the Trover Campus of the University of Louisville School of Medicine. This report described a significant decrease in utilization of emergency department and hospitalization services and improved functional status among free clinic patients in the 10 month period after they established care, compared to a similar period before free clinic care.

Ellett and colleagues conducted a study to examine patient satisfaction with the services provided by a student-run free clinic and found a high level of overall satisfaction with most aspects of care at the clinic. The areas in which patients expressed the least satisfaction were clinic hours and wait time, while patients were highly satisfied with laboratory services, staff friendliness, amount of time being interviewed, and depth of explanations. Based on study results students and faculty at the clinic began making changes in clinic services and structures.

Given the substantial role and potential impact of free clinic services, it is important to continue to assess the quality of their services, including the use of patient satisfaction measures. The current study, conducted at HCCC, replicates the work by Ellett and colleagues but over a longer period of time with a larger number of patients. We also took this opportunity to allow representatives of students, staff, and faculty to provide their perspectives.

## DESCRIPTION OF THE FREE CLINIC

The Hopkins County Community Clinic (HCCC) was founded in 2004 to serve the working, uninsured, low income citizens of this western Kentucky county. In 2008, care was extended to the adjacent county of Webster utilizing the same clinic site in Madisonville. A single evening session each week (the "Cardinal Clinic') is staffed by medical students from the University of Louisville Trover Campus (ULTC), supervised on-site by volunteer local physicians. The ULTC Dean serves as the medical director for this effort. In addition, there is a daytime session staffed by a paid, part-time nurse practitioner. Other part-time paid staff includes a director, a patient representative who serves as medication coordinator, a receptionist, and nurses. A volunteer community board sets policy for the clinic. The clinic is established as a 501 (c) 3 nonprofit organization, and receives funding from United Way, city and county governments, private businesses, individuals, civic organizations, and an annual charity fund-raiser.

New patients complete a complex financial assessment with considerable help from the staff. Upon verification of income below 185% of the federal poverty level, work status, Hopkins or Webster County residence, and lack of any private or governmental medical insurance, the patient is scheduled for a new patient appointment. This same documentation is needed for the forms required for pharmaceutical companies' patient assistance programs, facilitating the provision of free medications prescribed at the first and subsequent visits. Basic laboratory and imaging studies along with limited specialty consultations are provided to HCCC patients at no charge by the Trover Health System.

The Cardinal Clinic medical director completes regular chart reviews on all patient encounters by students, and these are discussed in a monthly group session with all the participating third-year students at a regular "Dean's Hour." Students prepare and update clinical protocols for common conditions including hypertension, diabetes, and hyperlipidemia. At the group sessions, adherence to the protocols and required exceptions are discussed. This review serves as a performance improvement (PI) opportunity and allows the students to learn this process early in their clinical training.

Fourth-year medical students have the opportunity to take a formal elective credit course using the clinic as a PI laboratory. The student reviews some practical PI publications, identifies a clinic process that could be better, and then prepares a short report with suggestions for improvement that is shared with the clinic staff.

## METHODS

From March through June, 2010, a survey was completed by patients seen in the student-directed portion of the HCCC. Blank surveys were given to the patients by the students, who introduced the survey with the following script: "We would really like you to tell us how we're doing. Please complete this brief survey and put it in the box at the patient representative's desk on your way out." This was a drop-box with a slot that required that the survey be folded in half, so anonymity was ensured. At the end of each clinic session, the patient representative wrote on the back of each survey the date and a unique sequential case ID number.

Prior to beginning the survey, the five third-year medical students most involved in the free clinic met with the clinic medical director (WJC) and Executive Director (MAK) and predicted potential correlations among the variables included in the survey. Then they individually and anonymously answered the questions on the survey concerning perceptions of the service provided by the clinic as they predicted the patients would. The students also at this same time provided their perceptions of their own health and the degree to which they were in control of their own health. At the initiation of the survey, the students predicted that the patients would 1) be generally appreciative and report most services to be better than expected, 2) be less positive about the number of hours the clinic was open and the availability of tests and x-rays, 3) report somewhat worse health than one year ago, and 4) report that the control over their health is mostly in others' hands.

## RESULTS

Survey results were entered first into an Excel spreadsheet, with complete data for 108 surveys. Thirty nine surveys were incomplete (27%) and were not included in further analysis. The mean age of respondents was 44.9 while the mean number of prior visits to the clinic was 4.5. Of the respondents, 77 percent where white and 59 percent were female. For comparison, the database used to manage the Patient Assistance Program for free medications for all clinic patients over the last 4 years showed 66% were female and 82 % white. The ages in this database were collected only in brackets, but 49% were in the 45-64 year-old range, and 92% were in the 25-64 year-old range.

The range of responses to the nine questions about clinic processes showed the vast majority were satisfied with all aspects. Six percent indicated that the time taken to get an appointment needed improvement, and 14% said the time spent in the waiting room was too long. Nine percent stated that the clinic hours should be expanded and nine percent thought the delay in getting medication refills was too long.

Overall, thirty percent of patient respondents indicated a need for improvement in at least one of the nine areas, while eighty percent of the students saw room for improvement in some area. In the specific area of the care provided by students, only two percent of patients stated a need for improvement and twenty percent of students indicated improvement was needed. Twenty one percent of patient respondents stated that their general health was worse than it was a year ago while no students chose this option. In the area of health control, twelve percent of patients stated that control was mostly or only in others hands and none of the students indicated this to be true about themselves.

Twenty-nine patients made written comments. Most of these comments were positive, such as, "Don't change anything." "You all are greatly appreciated." "Thanks for all you do for us," and "to me you all are very good at what you do." "I'm glad that you all are here." There were a few negative comments that were very specific in nature like a need for a very quiet waiting room because of a chronic medical condition or just a larger waiting room.

After the descriptive analysis was complete, the data were entered into SPSS and chi-square and ANOVA analysis was performed. The first analysis showed a trend of patient response based on gender and number of previous clinic visits, but on closer review there was too little variation in any of the cells to allow for valid quantitative analysis.

## DISCUSSION

Overall, 99% of the patients surveyed were satisfied with their care, comparing well to the 98% reported by Ellett et al (3). Thirty per cent felt that some aspect of free clinic care could still be improved, with the wait time and the limited hours of clinic operation being the two primary concerns. However, our patients were more satisfied with those issues than those reported by Ellett et al, with that report citing 36% concerned about wait time and 41% about limited clinic hours, where our numbers were 14% and 9%, respectively. The students working in the clinic predictably saw more opportunities for improvement. However, only 2% of patient respondents saw a need for change in the care provided by the students, a reflection of their sincere appreciation for the quality of the students' volunteer activities.

There are aspects of the study design that may limit the generalizability of our findings. The patients surveyed may not have been representative of all of the Cardinal Clinic patients. However, the non-response rate of 27% is actually better than that reported in most surveys and some of these were actually probably repeat visits by the same patient during the study period. Because of the anonymous nature of the data collection, there is no way to determine if a blank or mostly blank form represents a patient declining to answer, inability to read, or a patient choosing not to repeat answering the survey. Our patient representative was trained to offer to read the form to anyone who hesitated or who "forgot their glasses," but this may still have been an issue. The demographics of those surveyed matched closely to the overall free clinic population, further supporting that respondents did mirror the entire clinic population.

## STUDENT PERCEPTIONS

The number of students participating in the free clinic program at the Trover Campus is small but growing. Forty five students have participated since 2004. Five students from the class of 2011 participated in staffing and running HCCC last year, compared to twelve students from the class of 2012 involved in the clinic this year. Given the growing numbers, we hope to produce a more systematic study of student benefits from participation in the future.

Nevertheless, anecdotally our students have always cited the free clinic as one of the most important learning experiences of their third and fourth years of medical school on our campus. The lessons they glean from participation in the clinic fall into two broad categories: practicing the nuts and bolts of patient care and understanding the differences in care for those who have full access to the healthcare system and those who do not.

As with all medical school rotations, the free clinic is supervised by an attending physician. But the free clinic model allows the student greater autonomy and responsibility during the entire process of patient care, from initial presentation to making a plan and documenting the visit. Students note that they learn efficiency, thoroughness, and clarity in documentation during free clinic participation to an extent that they do not experience in other rotations. Unlike other rotations, the free clinic experience also encourages students to participate in follow-up and continuity of care, giving them a chance to understand first-hand the challenges of patient adherence to treatment plans or failure of treatment and, on the other hand, the progress that can be made in tackling chronic conditions.

The limited access to laboratory, imaging, and specialist referral for free clinic patients is an additional lesson in considering alternative diagnostic tools and treatment options for patients. More importantly, perhaps, these limitations offer a glimpse of the range of challenges faced by healthcare in the United States. For some, limited access may mean a delay in important diagnostic studies or a complete lack of certain kinds of preventative services that are routinely recommended to all patients. Working with limited resources is a reality for these patients and their physicians, who must determine where to allocate limited pro bono offers of specialist consultations or CT scans. On the other hand, the practice of medicine with limited resources also contrasts with the more frequent use of advanced imaging or specialist referral that medical students see daily in other areas of the hospital or clinic. Students have the chance to learn to question the necessity of ordering these diagnostic tools when perhaps a good history and physical have already determined the next steps in care.

Above all, the free clinic experience gives students the chance to decide what kind of patient advocate they will become. Students see patients who are working but uninsured, who are often challenging in their complexity and difficulty complying with treatment, and who often present a range of psychosocial challenges along with their medical needs. These encounters offer students a clear illustration of the kind of energy and compassion that is required for good patient care for those most in need.

## STAFF PERSPECTIVE

The impact of the more frequent hands-on work by the students in our clinic is significant and has established a remarkable response to volunteerism that they can take with them throughout their career. When new M-3 students come into the program, they are sometimes a little timid about approaching and assessing patients, but after just a few sessions, they quickly become engaged with the care of the patients. They follow the care of the patients and some students actually take on the continued care of specific patients through their M-4 year.

The impact of this clinic is just as great for the patients. Many patients have told us stories of how they had gone without medical care or much needed medication due to financial constraints. Many times their chronic illnesses, left untreated, have put them in a crisis situation. We receive many positive comments and letters of appreciation from our patients telling us of their gratefulness and benefit of having this clinic. This clinic also provides a unique opportunity for a true partnership with the whole community. As the director approaches community leaders for support, the benefits are immediately obvious. For instance, a mayor knows that the spouse of a city employee who can't afford family health insurance coverage can get quality care at our free clinic. Easy and enthusiastic support generally follows any request.

## FACULTY PERSPECTIVE

Most adult primary care physicians in the 2 counties served by the free clinic take their turn supervising the care that the students provide. It is a positive experience to see their enthusiasm for patient care, and the responsibility of the faculty for the night is limited, knowing that the medical director is responsible for all follow-up issues. The volunteer physicians get to see the students mature as clinicians, becoming efficient and confident as they become patient advocates. From a leadership perspective, the student directors accepted feedback and have implemented new processes to decrease the time the patient spends in the waiting room.

Students, with faculty support, have also have learned to manage patients via telephone to spread out return visits so as to open up new patient appointment slots to decrease the wait time until a new patient slot is available.

## FURTHER STUDY

More patient satisfaction data will be collected after the performance improvements listed above have been fully implemented. More formal studies of student satisfaction and performance, along with careful chart review of the adherence to the clinical protocols are needed. In addition, more attention to the study of the health locus of control aspect in free clinic patients is indicated. Medical student-directed free clinics provide an ideal laboratory to measure the powerful effects of service learning.

## ACKNOWLEDGEMENT

We express our sincere appreciation for the cooperation of our patients, the support of the free clinic board, and the hard work of all the clinic volunteers and paid staff. The Trover Health System provided uncompensated lab tests, imaging, and some consultation for these patients. Many pharmaceutical companies provided the free medications from their assistance programs for the needy, and the University of Louisville Trover Campus (ULTC) provided support for data collection and analysis. A special thanks goes to Steve Fricker, ULTC Director of Student Affairs/Rural Health who supervised all survey development, data entry and data analysis.

# COMMUNITY ENGAGEMENT: SERVICE LEARNING AS THE TOUCHSTONE

*Dr. Crump says that service learning is the only experience that allows students to learn the concepts of community medicine. As he built the campus career pathways programs that would earn national awards for educational innovation, service learning was the matrix. His campus would also earn a national award for community engagement. The following article is an example. It describes a community effort that he says is the most fun he has at work.*

Crump WJ, Fisher SM, Fricker RS. Community Service as Learning Laboratory: A Report of Six Years of a Rural Community-Academic Partnership.
Journal of the Kentucky Medical Association. 2014; 122: 131-136.

## ABSTRACT

Service learning is an important strategy to interest medical students in underserved areas. Urban medical schools can provide the resources to create quality service learning opportunities, but doing this in rural areas is more difficult. The authors report 6 years of experience with the provision of free school physical exams in two rural counties by students based at the rural University of Louisville Trover Campus (ULTC), serving 402 school children across 6 summers. Students worked alongside health department and school staff. Evaluations included those from community staff, patients, parents, and the students. Significant health issues were found in 9.7% of the children. "Teach back" evaluations showed that the children understood the anticipatory guidance provided, and parents and community staff feedback was uniformly positive. Staff comments clearly demonstrated ownership of the process and appreciation of the students' efforts. Students also expressed confidence in their developing medical skills and a new understanding of health disparities, barriers, and health belief issues encountered. Compared to students not participating in the program, 22% vs 9% later chose family medicine residencies and 32% vs 10% chose rural practice. Rural regional campuses can be a resource to support a service learning laboratory and ensuring community involvement in every aspect can result in a sense of ownership and pride for what can become a self-sustaining community-academic partnership. Future efforts should include more comprehensive evaluation methods and attempt to include health students from other disciplines.

## PROBLEM

The shortage of rural physicians is a significant problem for ensuring access to care for the 19% of Americans who live in small towns. Recent reports have supported the affinity model, where students from rural areas who are trained in more rural settings are more likely to choose rural practice. An important aspect of rural physician recruitment and retention is the strong connection these physicians feel to their communities, and the understanding of these issues can be increased by planned didactic activities during medical school in an urban environment. However, experiential learning in a community setting is generally considered the most powerful method for cementing this connection in what is often termed community medicine. A recent comprehensive review found 57 articles that addressed medical education in community service learning environments. They found five themes, including that service learning often: 1) is organized around concerns expressed by the community itself, and not only by well-meaning outside interests; 2) is consciously designed to provide important benefit both to the community and the participating students, often providing a tangible service such as health screenings or health education; 3) includes explicit opportunities for students to discover health disparities, health care barriers, and social determinants of health; 4) includes experiential learning of the details of health systems function, including funding mechanisms and the value of interdisciplinary teams; and, 5) has cultural competency as a stated goal, including understanding of unique local health beliefs.

Most of these reports are from urban underserved environments because the resources of the urban-based medical school are necessary to ensure a quality learning experience. A few reports have shown that a similar effort in rural areas can improve student attitudes toward working with underserved populations. As more rural regional medical school campuses are established, this provides an opportunity to use medical school resources to provide a quality rural service learning environment.

We report here a summer preclinical program structured around a community-based service learning project including premedical and preclinical medical students based from a small, regional rural medical school campus. The University of Louisville Trover Campus (ULTC) was established in 1998 and is located in a town of 20,000 in the western Kentucky coalfields, approximately 150 miles southwest of the parent campus in Louisville. It serves as a regional clinical campus where 8-12 students move each year after their first two years in Louisville, completing all of their M-3 and M-4 rotations in the Madisonville area.

## APPROACH

Early versions of this program began in 1998. The Preclinical Student Screening Team (PSST) project began in 2006 with rising M-2 medical students receiving a 3-day tutorial on the screening history and physical exam and then performing school physicals in adjacent underserved counties by invitation of county leaders. Preclinical students work with premedical college students in the Trover Rural Scholar (TRS) program. The physicals are supervised by one faculty family medicine physician (WJC). One author (SF) served as a premedical student for three summers and then as a preclinical student. The curriculum for the 3 week program also includes rural physician precepting and group sessions on clinical reasoning based on a case discussion, with each preclinical student leading a group of premedical students.

Prior to 2006, community service activities for the ULTC preclinical programs included participating in a multi-site statewide program managed from Louisville. The western Kentucky sites were chosen based on underserved status, but there were no members of the western Kentucky communities on the planning group. The students enjoyed these activities, but the patient volume was very low, with about 3-5 patients seen per half-day session. As PSST was planned, community health councils formed by an earlier ULTC student activity were used as informal focus groups.

The community health councils, lead principally by county health department and school staff, expressed a strong need for state-required school physicals and sports physicals. There was already a large, station-based event to provide free sports physicals held once per year 30 minutes away in the regional referral center in Madisonville, the site of the ULTC campus. For these sports physicals and the required school physicals, only one local provider was available in each county who could do these exams at any other time. The councils from both counties reported that many of the most needy families in their areas could not get their children to the local providers when scarce appointment times were available nor to the annual event 30 minutes away. The result was that the first few days of the new school year and the sports practice time were disrupted by students being removed from important activities until the required exams could be completed.

The two counties were 98% and 93% white, with populations of 10,000 and 14,000, and 17% and 16% of persons below poverty level, respectively (Kentucky-wide, this number is 18%.) Both counties are considered Health Professional Shortage Areas (HPSA).

Working with community stake-holders, dates and times were established for the PSST sessions, and flyers were posted around the community several weeks before the first session. In addition, the school-based Family Resource and Youth Service Centers (FRYSC) mailed a notice to each rising 6th grader's home and also notified families individually known to be in need. A community panel traveled to the UTLC campus before the community activities began to discuss topics that are important to their individual county. Immediately after the panel and continuing for the next 3 weeks, teams of 2 students each conducted community key informant interviews to learn more details.

The preclinical medical students and premedical students worked closely together to plan the sessions. They collected anticipatory guidance props and pamphlets about safe sex, smoking, alcohol, drugs, sunscreen, and bicycle, car, and ATV safety.

After the medical student examination, the attending physician would then talk with the patient, repeat the physical examination, and document any needed further evaluations. Referrals for consultation or testing were explained to the parents and communicated to on-site health department or FRYSC staff, who then took a copy of the form to the appropriate school nurse to coordinate all subsequent care. Each child received individual anticipatory guidance counseling from the premedical student.

At the conclusion of the counseling, the premedical student conducted a "teach-back" evaluation to judge the child's knowledge of the topics addressed and scored the child's understanding on a Likert scale. The parent's and community staff evaluation consisted of questions about the students, the physical examination, and overall experience. The answers were also based on a Likert scale, all recorded anonymously. Once all of the physical examinations were completed and all families had left the site, staff, faculty and students discussed the day's process, abnormalities, and required referrals.

The students completed a detailed county assessment report that was presented to ULTC staff and county representatives at the conclusion of the program. The report was based on available statistics, common abnormal findings, and key informant interviews.

At the end of the program, the students completed an anonymous program evaluation, rating how well each component of the program accomplished the goals as well as their enjoyment of each.

We calculated and reported simple descriptive frequencies, percentages, means, and standard deviations and tested with chi square to examine the relationship between participation and subsequent specialty choice and location of practice. For Likert scale data, we calculated and reported simple frequencies and percentages.

We coded the ULSOM residency match list for the classes of 2001 through 2010 as Family Medicine or all other. We also coded ULSOM graduates from the classes of 2001 through 2006 (who would have established practice) to the American Medical Association (AMA) Physician Master File as metropolitan/non-metropolitan, using RUCC codes for location of practice.

After data were coded utilizing Microsoft Excel 2003, they were imported into SPSS v. 20 (IBM Corp, Armonk, NY). We then used Chi-square to determine significance. The Trover Health System Institutional Review Board determined that this activity was exempt.

## OUTCOMES

Over the six summers, 402 school physicals were performed, with 39% also including a sports physical. Follow-up was suggested in 39 (9.7%). The parent evaluation was completed by 392 parents and 26 community staff members and were uniformly positive At the end of the program, 81% of the students said that some aspect of PSST was their favorite part of the program.

Previous participants in some version of this program chose family medicine residencies more frequently (9 of 40 for 22%) than all ULSOM graduates who did not participate (116 of 1311 for 9%), p<.01. In addition, more previous participants chose rural practice (8 of 25 for 32%) than all ULSOM graduates who did not participate (75 of 766 for 10%), p <.01.

The program accomplished the goals using a community service learning laboratory as the focus. The effort was organized around concerns expressed by community members, and this explains much of its success. It also provided tangible benefits to the community participants in the form of a completed school evaluation with specific recommendations provided to both parents and school-based staff who were clearly tasked with the continuity needed to implement the suggestions. The students also clearly benefited, both with new confidence in their medical skills and new understanding of the function of health department and school-based services.

At the de-briefing sessions, the faculty facilitator often asked the community staff why the project seems to be so successful year to year. The answers spoke to ownership, with the FRYSC director at one session remarking that getting almost two-thirds of "our" rising 6th graders through "our" process and knowing they were now ready to start school was a "real blessing." The health department nursing director said: "It's truly a unique relationship, and incredibly constructive. We [the health department staff] learn from the medical students, and they learn from us. The medical students and physicians are respectful and I think they respect public health even more now. All in all, the PSST is completely worth it. I think something like the PSST will always be needed."

## NEXT STEPS

The evaluation of this project was limited by the absence of more precise pre- and post- measures of student attitudes and skills. The measures gave good qualitative feedback that the methods were accomplishing the goals, but more precise measures would be helpful in future efforts. Also, we did not ask specific questions of the students pre-and post-involvement that could have proven our impression that they had improved attitudes about working in underserved areas and working in community-based environments. Our impression is supported by a significantly greater proportion of participants in some version of this program choosing family medicine and subsequent rural practice, but it is possible that self- selection of the students to this program may explain some of that difference. Retention in rural practice may be a better measure of community connection than initial practice choice, and that will require our continued tracking of the practice site of participants in our programs, and we now do that on an annual basis. Generalizability of our findings is also limited to similar communities and similar students.

Our students got a good opportunity to work with established community professionals outside of medicine, but a more complete interdisciplinary experience could include students in these disciplines working alongside the medical students. The rural location and distance to other health education facilities will make this a challenge, but could be an important complement to the existing program.

We recommend that those planning similar activities follow Hunt's five elements prospectively. For those interested in producing more community-minded physicians, a comment from one student is a good summary:

"PSST is a unique, real-world application of what we learn. There could never be a stronger motivator for academic success than the patients. Just having a role during the screenings challenged me to do well in school … so I can give back more someday."

## ACKNOWLEDGEMENT

Without the tireless efforts of all our community partners, this program would not have been successful. West Kentucky AHEC was also an active partner. Pam Carter managed every detail of this program including tracking outcomes. Craig Ziegler, biostatistician with ULSOM, provided statistical consultations on the analysis.

# GETTING DOCS TO SMALL TOWNS: AN ACCELERATED CURRICULUM

*As the campus matured and graduates began returning to small towns to practice, the gap still widened as more rural docs retired. An essay in the premier academic medical journal caught Dr. Crump's eye. The author made the point that the vast majority of admitted medical students were from urban wealthy families. The other group of young people, those most likely to choose small town practice, were intimidated by the cost and extended training duration required to become a doctor. To allow these capable young students to choose medicine, the author proposed shortening the time required in medical school, thereby also decreasing the tuition cost by 25%. At about the same time, reports highlighted such a program that was finally approved by the medical school accrediting body (LCME) at Texas Tech in Lubbock. Dr. Crump pitched the idea to the new dean in Louisville who had a heart for the urban underserved, and the race was on. The Trover Campus became the home of the second such accelerated medical school track in the U.S. There are now over 40 such programs, and Dr. Crump brings his historical perspective to the consortium supporting this innovation. The two articles that follow summarize the effort at the Trover Campus.*

Crump WJ, Wiegman David L, Fricker RS. An Accelerated Track to Rural Practice: An Option to Complete Medical School in Three Years. Journal of the Kentucky Academy of Family Physicians. Winter 2013; 78: 20-22.

## BACKGROUND

America's rural areas are severely underserved, with 20% of the U. S population living in small towns, but only 9% of doctors practicing there. Family doctors distribute more evenly, with 22% practicing outside of urban areas. The most effective methods for addressing this need are to facilitate medical school admission by students from rural areas and train them outside of urban areas. The effectiveness of this strategy is limited by the small numbers of successful rural applicants. Pipeline programs facilitating academic preparation of rural students are promising, and once the students from small towns matriculate, they do as well as their urban counterparts in medical school. However, many rural students cite the length of training and the costs as significant barriers to their even considering medical school.

One strategy to address this issue is to shorten medical school, saving an entire year of tuition while allowing entry into a paying residency position earlier. The idea reached national academic attention in 2006 with an essay by the Editor of Academic Medicine that made the case that financial barriers may exclude many students coming from families of modest means, the most likely to choose rural practice, from consideration of medical school. A companion editorial in the same journal suggested specific methods to shorten medical training to lessen these financial barriers. In the academic setting, this option was discussed among the Dean's staff at the University of Louisville and the leadership of the Trover rural regional medical school campus with options for implementation considered. When Texas Tech announced in 2009 that they had received LCME approval to institute such a track, the planning process began in earnest.

A formal application was submitted to the LCME, with final approval in March, 2011 to begin the rural option based at the Trover rural campus in Madisonville for this accelerated track, with consideration for an urban underserved option to be developed later. The track was designated the

Rural Medicine Accelerated Track (RMAT). The structure did not change the basic science M-1 and M-2 years, except that the two-month summer break after the M-1 year and the one-month break after the M-2 year were incorporated into rural clinical rotations. These additions and allocation of all M-3 elective time to RMAT met the requirement for 130 weeks of medical education between matriculation and beginning residency. The decision was made not to tie the RMAT to any specific residency program. The decision was also made to allow students to enter the track in the spring of the M-2 year rather than at admission. Those intending to apply for the RMAT would have participated in the summer activities prior to this decision point, and either the student or the track director could suggest that the 4-year option was better for this individual student. Waiting until this time provided a track record of both academic performance in medical school and demonstrated commitment to rural practice, making success more likely for the RMAT student. The first 2 students in the pilot began their first rural rotation (RMAT-1) in summer, 2012.

## ISSUES WITH IMPLEMENTATION

For those considering adding an accelerated track option, this six-year planning process taught us some lessons. First, institutional commitment is key. The ULSOM Dean initiated the process, and tasked the Senior Dean for Education at the main campus to obtain input and advice from all key academic leaders. A 16 month process then ensued including multiple meetings of the champions of the idea with all leaders of primary care on the main campus. A separate meeting was held with key family medicine faculty, ultimately resulting in endorsement by the chair. With the current interest in extending FM residency training beyond 3 years, some saw shortening medical school as an attractive option. Others expressed concern that if the accelerated curriculum were confined to those seeking a FM residency, the prestige of the discipline in the academic center could be damaged. When all concerns were addressed, the final proposal was submitted to the LCME.

Secondly, there is the issue of recruitment of students. Initially, we thought it may be difficult to find many medical students motivated to undertake the RMAT. It requires a mature student who is sure of specialty choice and comfortable with the high probability of matching with a regional residency. Subsequently, several students have indicated that the opportunity to "just move once" from Louisville and spend the last 4 years in Madisonville is very attractive to them. For students concerned with mounting debt, the opportunity to save one year of tuition cost while earning a PG-1 income is also very attractive. This is a net gain of about $100,000 in that year.

The issue of limitation of residency choice was also a concern. Most accelerated programs assume that their graduates will stay in the residency associated with the campus, but some do not. The accelerated graduates clearly have an advantage in their local residency, as they are "known quantities." If the student decides during the M-3 year that he/she wants to match elsewhere, even potentially in a different specialty, he/she maybe at a competitive disadvantage.

From a Residency Program Director perspective, these students' USMLE step 2 scores will not be available as the match list is completed and their accelerated clinical experience may be poorly understood. Directors interviewed reported that when considering accelerated graduates they will place more emphasis on clinical grades and shelf exam scores from the M-3 year, and one indicated he would place more emphasis on USMLE step one scores. The RMAT graduate who chooses a very competitive FM program outside of the region or in another specialty may not be viewed as positively as a graduate from a U.S. school with a traditional four-year curriculum. Potential RMAT participants are advised of this in advance of their decision to participate, and adequate time is provided for interviewing at other programs in the fall of the M-3 year. If their career plans change significantly, they have the option of returning to the 4-year curriculum.

## CONCLUSION

With heightened awareness of the need for more primary care doctors and the focus on maldistribution of physicians, the timing is right for innovative methods of producing more rural physicians. RMAT may be a path for rural students from families of modest means who otherwise may have chosen another career to complete medical school and practice near home.

**Crump WJ, Jessup, Ashley. Early Experience with an Accelerated Medical School Track to Rural Practice. Journal of Kentucky Medical Association. 2015; 113: 55-57.**

Many rural students cite length of training and cost as barriers to attempting medical school1. One old strategy that re-entered the national discussion again 8 years ago is to shorten medical school, saving an entire year of tuition while allowing entry into a paying residency position earlier2-3. To accomplish this, The University of Louisville Trover rural regional medical school campus (ULTC) proposed a structure modified from the Texas Tech schedule and a pilot program was approved by the LCME in 2011. RMAT students are a subset of the 12 students admitted to the ULSOM each year knowing that they will do all their clinical rotations at the Trover Campus in Madisonville, a town of 20, 000 that is 150 miles southwest of Louisville.

The track was designated the Rural Medicine Accelerated Track (RMAT). The structure did not change the basic science M-1 and M-2 years in Louisville, except that the two-month summer break after the M-1 year and the one-month break after the M-2 year were incorporated into rural clinical rotations. These additions and allocation of all M-3 elective time to RMAT met the requirement for 130 weeks of medical education between matriculation and beginning residency. The decision was made not to tie the RMAT to any specific residency program and to allow students to enter the track in the spring of the M-2 year rather than at admission. The six-year planning process for RMAT has been described previously. The outcome we report here is the feedback on this implementation phase after our first RMAT student graduated, from a ten-item structured questionnaire that was sent to key administrative leaders.

The student perspective was that rural shadowing during college made the decision to choose RMAT easier. This student had both worked in a rural doctor's office and participated in the Trover College Rural Scholar summer program during college. The opportunity to wait until spring of the M-2 year to enter RMAT allowed confidence to develop that it was a good match and that the student could be successful on an accelerated schedule. Doing a detailed rural practice assessment near home after the M-1 year solidified the student's plans, and a rotation at the rural regional campus during this same summer served as an "audition."

Maintaining the full 5 week step one study period that all students had after the M-2 year was important. Doing a rotation at the rural campus' free clinic soon after the M-2 year allowed for beginning continuity with patients before the rest of the class, maximizing what was learned from this longitudinal experience. Scheduling USMLE step 2 CK and CS during the M-3 year was daunting, but performance on them was not. The student felt well prepared, and the 17 point increment between step 1 and step 2 CK was actually higher than the mean increment reported at either campus when step 2 was taken during the M-4 year. Allowing RMAT students to interview widely and complete the match process ultimately increased the student's confidence in the decision to match at the residency in the same small town as the regional campus.

Although some program directors expressed concern that step 2 CK and CS results would not be known prior to submitting their match list, the student reported that most were genuinely interested in current and future RMAT students. In fact RMAT was an excellent talking point during interviews. Knowing that there was no time allowed for illness or academic difficulties was stressful, but knowing that at any point the student could revert to the four-year schedule was reassuring. The RMAT student didn't perceive working any harder than classmates, but preparing for step 2 CK and CS while on demanding M-3 rotations required commitment and efficiency.

The opportunity to wait until spring of the M-2 year to enter RMAT allowed the selection committee to have confidence that it was a good match. By this time 3 semesters of medical school work were completed and the rural dean had feedback from a rural 4-week experience and 4 weeks personal experience working with the student at the rural campus. Some accelerated programs choosing students prior to admission tend to select those with stronger college academic performance as a "safe bet." This might actually exclude some rural students who can be "late bloomers" and do well in medical school.

From the program directors' perspective, there was genuine concern that a match list decision had to be made prior to knowing the step 2 CK and CS scores and with grades from only three clinical M-3 rotations. Program directors were reassured by the careful description of RMAT in the student's MSPE (Dean's letter) and that there had been a careful "audition" and "vetting" process that included 3 other rigorous clinical rotations prior to beginning the M-3 year. They also looked more closely at step one scores. For the program that is based in the town with the rural Trover Campus, the decision to rank was much easier because the student had done a 6-week acting intern rotation on their very busy inpatient service and was a "known quantity." They also said that the required commitment and efficiency of any student completing the demanding RMAT schedule was a good predictor of success in residency. The directors also said that allowing the student to interview as widely as they liked was good for the student, but that the "home" program would clearly have both a recruiting advantage and more confidence in ranking the student among other strong candidates.

It's time for innovative methods of producing more rural physicians. RMAT may allow rural students who otherwise may have chosen another career to complete medical school and practice near home.

## DISTINCTIVE FEATURES OF THE ULTC RMAT:

1. All clinical experience is in very small rural towns across all 3 years.
2. Admission to the track occurs during the M-2 year, not at admission to medical school.
3. At least one full 4-week rotation occurs near student's hometown.
4. An early start in a rural free clinic provides a full 12 month longitudinal experience.
5. Students are not limited to any residency program or specialty.
6. Students enter the match process during the M-3 (final) year.
7. Return to the standard 4-year curriculum is easy if personal or academic issues arise.

Acknowledgements: We thank the almost 40 faculty from the primary care disciplines at ULSOM who worked with us to establish this innovative program as well as the rural physicians who opened their practices to RMAT students and completed the very detailed evaluation instruments. A special thanks goes to Dr. David Wiegman, Vice Dean for Academic Affairs, Dr. Toni Ganzel, Dean of the ULSOM who was Senior Associate Dean for Students and Academic Affairs at the time RMAT began, and Steve Fricker, the ULTC Director of Student Health/Rural Affairs. These three did the required detailed work necessary to prepare a successful proposal for LCME approval.

# THE PROOF IS IN THE RESULTS: OUTCOMES

*As the Trover Campus began to draw national attention, a key question was asked. The vastly higher percentage of their graduates choosing small town practice was undeniable, but was it just that the campus attracted those already from small towns with an early interest in family medicine? Connecting with a biostatistician on the Louisville campus and with tedious data management, Dr. Crump set out to do something not published previously. Using statistical methods to control for these two predilections for rural practice, his team showed definitively that the Trover Campus experience added significantly to the likelihood that graduates would ultimately choose small town practice. His campus received another national award for educational innovation.*

Crump WJ, Fricker RS, Ziegler CH, Wiegman DL. Increasing the Rural Physician Workforce: A Potential Role for Small Rural Medical School Campuses. The Journal of Rural Health. 2016; 32(3):254-259.

## ABSTRACT

### PURPOSE

To address the issue of physician maldistribution, some medical schools have rural-focused efforts, and many more are in the planning or early implementation stage. The best duration and structure of the rural immersion experience are unclear, and the relative effects of rural upbringing and rural training on subsequent rural practice choice are often difficult to determine.

## METHODS

To determine the effect of adding a rural clinical campus to our school, we analyzed the variables of rural upbringing, demographics, family medicine residency choice, and campus participation using a multivariate model for association with rural practice choice. We included graduates from the classes of 2001-2008 from both campuses (urban and rural) in the analysis.

## FINDINGS

We found similar associations to those reported previously of rural upbringing (OR=2.67 [1.58-4.52]) and family medicine residency (OR=5.08 [2.88-8.98]) with rural practice choice. Even controlling for these 2 variables, participation in the full 2 years at the rural clinical campus showed the strongest association (OR=5.46 [2.61-11.42]). All 3 associations were significant at $P < .001$, and no other variables were significant.

## CONCLUSIONS

We conclude that the investment of resources in our rural campus may add an increment to rural practice choice beyond the established associations with rural upbringing and family medicine residency. The decision of practice site choice is complex, and collaborative studies that include data from several schools with differently structured rural exposures, including those with rural clinical campuses, are needed.

## PURPOSE

Without more emphasis on programs that produce more rural physicians, simply increasing the number of medical school graduates is unlikely to address the problem of maldistribution of physicians. The affinity model proposes that when a student who is from a rural area is trained in less urbanized areas, that student is more likely to return to a small town to practice. More recent studies have supported this model. The programs showing the most success in placing graduates into rural practice include preferential admission of rural students, financial assistance, active mentoring, and a rural immersion experience. Programs that attempt to optimize the affinity model with a longer rural immersion experience can be challenged by limitations of graduate educational resources in rural areas. Without an adequate "dose" of rural experience during medical school, the risk is that rural students with an initial affinity for rural practice then experience "urban disruption," becoming attracted to big-city life during their medical education, which is typically in urban areas. More recently, some medical schools have placed clinical campus resources in smaller towns to try to take full advantage of the affinity model.

Most rural-focused special programs allow students to self-select and therefore each step in training pathways can potentially magnify the effect of the affinity model, but this makes isolating the effect of the program itself difficult. The unanswered question is the duration and structure of rural experience options that will best attract those with a rural affinity and maximize the likelihood of choice of rural practice. A longer rural experience would presumably be more effective, but it is also more expensive and potentially disruptive to the household of a student whose primary residence is in the urban site of their medical school. Established programs have rural experiences during the clinical years varying from 6 weeks to 4 months to 9 months. A longer immersion experience is provided by rural regional campuses, where the entire 2-year clinical experience is rural.

While all of these efforts have been successful in placing students into rural practice, it is difficult to determine how much of the practice choice was the result of the programs (nurture) and how much was rural upbringing (nature). This is an important rural health policy issue, as medical schools and state legislatures that are committed to producing more rural physicians must make decisions about focusing more on admissions (nature) or alternatively on rural programs (nurture), or both.

A previous report from our school done before our rural campus was established supported the nature aspect, but it cited a potential negative effect of nurture, noting that "The cultures of medical schools tend to socialize students toward specialty careers and urban practice location."

We have previously reported that graduates from our rural campus were 6 times more likely to choose rural practice than their classmates who attended our urban campus who had only a 6-week rotation in a rural area (55% vs 9%). With these data, however, we were not able to differentiate between nature and nurture.

In the current report we use an analysis that allows us to determine the relative association of nature and nurture in a large group of graduates from both campuses. Our hypothesis was that having the rural campus option provides an additional increment in rural practice choice beyond rural upbringing or specialty choice. We found no previous US reports that used multivariate analysis that included rural and main urban campus participation as a predictor of rural practice.

## METHOD

After completing their first 2 years of basic sciences in Louisville, 6-12 medical students moved to the Trover campus in Madisonville, a town of 20,000 that is 150 miles southwest of Louisville. Students were based within a rural integrated health system with a 400-bed hospital staffed by 80 physicians representing primary and secondary care specialties. The system also included 10 satellite clinics within a 30-minute drive that are in towns of 4,000 to 8,000 that host portions of clinical rotations. Students participated in the same classroom lectures as the Louisville-based students by simultaneous live video connection. All curriculum elements, teaching materials, and evaluation systems were identical at the 2 campuses. Clinical rotations on the Trover campus provided the opportunity for one-on-one learning with an experienced clinician preceptor. On some of the clinical rotations, a family medicine resident was on the teaching service as well. All M-3 students regardless of rotation met for small group problem-based learning sessions twice a month, facilitated by the Trover campus Associate Dean, and they participated in longitudinal care for their panel of patients in a community clinic. A longitudinal teaching skills program was in place to assist the community-based faculty in guiding the students through their required clerkships.

During the time period reported here, students indicated their interest in placement at the Trover campus during the fall of the M-2 year, visited the campus, and met with current students. All students who indicated interest were accepted. Some of these students had participated in pathways programs previously, and 68% were from rural backgrounds. For this report, it is important to note that this selection of clinical campus was done almost 2 years after the admission decision, which was independent of which clinical campus the student would ultimately choose. The only selection process was student self-selection, as all interested students were accepted. Shortly after the time period reported here, the decision was made to begin dedicated admissions to the Trover campus. The competitive selection process was moved to the point of application for admission, so the student is admitted with assignment to the Louisville or Madisonville campus.

We studied all graduates from both campuses from 2001 to 2008, using the American Medical Association (AMA) Physician Master File for location of practice based upon primary office address, at the level of unit record data, matched by name. Demographics were collected from the American Medical College Application Service admissions application. Graduation from a high school located in a town with a population of < 30,000 was the rural criterion used by our admissions office, and it was used as a surrogate measure for rural upbringing. We then matched practice site location to Rural Urban Continuum Codes (RUCC) and used non-metropolitan RUCC codes as a surrogate to identify rural/small town practice. The RUCC categorizes counties into 9 classifications, 3 as metro and 6 as non-metro. For this analysis, we used the 6 non-metro classifications as a proxy for rural practice. In Kentucky, 3 of the non-metro counties had urban populations of approximately 28,000, and the majority had towns of only 4,000-9,000.

## STATISTICAL ANALYSIS

We used standard multiple logistic regression to assess the impact of medical students' rural training on practice location while adjusting for demographic variables. First, we calculated frequencies and percentages to assess independent associations. For the multiple logistic regression models we present adjusted odds ratios (OR) with 95% confidence intervals, along with the Nagelkerke $R^2$. The outcome variable consisted of practice location (rural versus non-rural). Student training consisted of 2 groups: (a) standard campus only and (b) rural clinical campus. Demographic characteristics that were controlled for include rural upbringing, family medicine residency, gender, age, degree type (undergraduate science or non-science), and race. We used SAS version 9.3 (SAS Institute Inc., Cary, North Carolina) to analyze the data. All P values were 2-tailed. We set statistical significance by convention at $P < .05$.

## FINDINGS

Eleven hundred and twenty medical school graduates from 2001 to 2008 constituted the database. Practicing in a rural location occurred in only 7% of standard campus graduates, but the proportion increased to 45% of rural campus graduates. The adjusted OR indicate that choosing a rural practice location was significantly higher for graduates participating in the rural campus (OR=5.46) compared with standard program graduates. Rural practice location was significantly associated with having a rural upbringing (OR=2.67), as well as choosing a family medicine residency (OR=5.08). No other variables achieved significance. Nagelkerke $R2 = 0.14$ when rural upbringing and specialty choice were in the model, but it increased to 0.19 after rural training was added.

## DISCUSSION

As found in many previous reports, rural upbringing and choice of family medicine specialty showed a significant association with rural practice. However, controlling for those effects, graduating from the rural campus showed the strongest association. This is the first time that such an association has been reported in a US medical school. None of the demographic measures were significant.

Earlier reports from the Trover Campus showed that urban disruption occurred when all but 6 weeks of the clinical training was in Louisville. Even though 41% of the students attending the urban campus were from rural areas, only 9% chose rural practice. Here we show that some of that attrition may be prevented by training rural students at a rural clinical campus. In this previous report, family medicine career choice was also strongly associated with rural clinical campus (37% vs 8%), but our current data show that even controlling for family medicine choice, the rural campus still shows the strongest odds ratio.

## LIMITATIONS

Our data are from one medical school, so generalizability is limited. The inclusion of a large population, including all the graduates from both campuses for 8 years using unit record data rather than aggregate data, strengthens the analysis. We included most predictors that had been found valuable in earlier studies, but this list resulted in removal of 15% of the observations because of missing data. This is typical of most multivariate analyses that strive to include variables collected from different sources.

As with any educational effort that is not randomized, the students at both campuses were largely self-selected, so we cannot say that the curriculum or environment of the rural campus itself accounted for the increment in rural practice choice. We can say that students choosing the rural campus option were more likely to choose rural practice. If the rural campus is an attractive option to students most likely to choose rural practice, the rural programs offering such an option should send more graduates to rural practice. Although the differences are not large, a recent report showed exactly that, with most of the medical school programs at the top in terms of producing rural physicians being based at rural clinical campuses.

Although we conclude that the investment of resources in our rural campus as an option may have added an increment to rural practice choice, adding all the measured variables together only increased the predictive power of practice location to 19%. While this is within the range of previously published studies, it shows that individual student choice is quite complex and there may be important variables that are outside the scope of undergraduate medical educators. Our experience tells us that relationships made with significant others during medical school, and a potential spouse's upbringing and occupational needs, are important in future practice choice. Even with telecommuting becoming more routine, some occupations have limited options in a rural area.

We have reported previously that some rural students have particularly close family ties, and that even a difference in 2-3 hours' drive to reach family affects their choice of medical school campuses. So a rural student or spouse may choose to live in an urban area that is closer to rurally placed family rather than in a rural area that provides them an otherwise attractive employment opportunity at the other end of the state.

Other aspects of undergraduate and residency experience that may affect practice choice are also difficult to measure. Our experience is that early interaction with an enthusiastic faculty member in a sub-specialty may cause a student to choose a similar path, necessitating an urban practice choice later. Also, our report addresses only the medical school component, and residency location has been proven to be a powerful predictor of practice choice as well. Our data on the main campus graduates did not include the rurality of their residency program, which might have explained more of the variability in practice choice. We also did not have data on which graduates participated in rural loan repayment programs that may have explained more of the variance.

We have focused here on first practice choice, and longer-term retention in rural areas will be important. We continue to track each cohort after they enter practice, and we will reassess predictors of longer term retention when enough time has passed.

The numbers in some of the comparison categories in our analysis are small, but the statistical significance is strong even with these small groups. These small numbers are important in a practical sense, as many of the Kentucky counties that are currently classified as Health Professional Shortage Areas would be re-classified if only 1-2 physicians were to locate there. In this case and in many other predominantly rural states, small numbers matter.

## FUTURE RESEARCH NEEDS

It is important to know the best duration and characteristics of rural immersion that will have the optimum effect of facilitating rural practice choice among rural medical students. If one could randomize rural students to urban or rural campuses and perhaps even among varying durations and styles of rural immersions, the results would be most helpful. This is unlikely to happen, as medical education affords choices to students at many levels. Medical educators who work with students in rural environments are often convinced that simply spending 2 more years of a student's life in the context of a very small town has to increase their affinity for rural practice.16 Add to this that these students are learning in environments where most of their patients are like them in cultural and social dimensions should also increase this affinity. Further, all of their faculty and staff have also chosen to live and work in small towns, potentially adding to affinity through role modeling.

Rural medical educators are also invested in their curriculum, believing that longitudinal experiences, opportunities for commitment to service, and community engagement are keys to reinforcing rural affinity. But it also may be that successful rural programs are simply selecting the students who have already sufficiently decided that rural practice is for them. Slightly less rurally committed rural students who choose the urban campus may have ultimately chosen urban practice independent of the context or programming of the curriculum.

A key need is a reliable measure of rural affinity prior to practice choice and an insight into the campus choice process among rural students. If the 2 groups enter their clinical years with similar rural affinity and the rural-based group increases affinity while the urban-based group decreases, then perhaps more support for rural-based training is advisable. If the rural-based students choose the rural campus because it is rural, this would provide support that they were already sufficiently motivated and the rural campus would have little additional effect.

We have some information about reasons for campus choice from 54 students who initially indicated interest in our rural campus during their preclinical years. The group that maintained their interest and matriculated at the rural campus actually placed a much higher priority on one-to-one clinical training than they did on experiencing small town life. Those rural students choosing the urban clinical campus placed a higher priority on big city amenities and presence of a university. Another study of 36 preclinical rural students at an urban medical school campus showed that a year-long didactic rural medicine elective experience maintained, and on some items, significantly augmented positive opinions of rural practice.

Another key approach may be qualitative studies during residency training of those with rural roots as they are making the practice choice decision. An older study showed that feeling prepared for small-town living was more important for retention than actually the feeling of being prepared for the practice of medicine in a small town. Larger scale individual interviews or focus groups with senior residents and their spouses may provide more insight into the variance not yet explained by traditional demographic measures (nature) or educational exposure (nurture).

## CONCLUSION

As other medical schools work to implement programs to increase rural practice choice, our findings may be useful. Continuing admissions efforts including emphasis on rural upbringing and the known predictors of family medicine choice are supported by our data. In addition, a rural clinical campus may add to the number of those who choose a rural practice. A rural campus may also provide the host community with significant benefits from the financial investment made by a medical school, as well as potential positive effects on recruitment and retention of the campus graduates.

An important next step will be for schools that have various rural-focused efforts to pool their data and analyze unit record subsets to identify key aspects of the experience which are most important in influencing rural practice choice. We are working with other members of the National Rural Health Association Rural Medical Education Group and the Association of American Medical Colleges Group on Regional Medical Campuses to facilitate this collaboration including our data sets.

## ACKNOWLEDGMENT

The authors thank Pam Carter and Shelia Justice, Trover Campus, and Emily Carr, Office of Medical Education – Louisville Campus, for their many hours of data retrieval and entry.

# DEVELOPING A PROFESSIONAL IDENTITY CURRICULUM

*As the Trover Campus curriculum and schedules of the pathways programs and clinical rotations settled and became routinized, Dr. Crump himself felt unsettled. His students at all levels were excelling as measured by traditional scores and going on to success in residency training and subsequently choosing small town practice. During the 2013-2015 years, many of his graduates chose to stay in Madisonville to complete their family medicine residency. As faculty, he had regular close interactions with them in obstetrics and when precepting them as they saw their office patients. He noticed something troubling. Many of these young physicians had morphed from idealistic, compassionate individuals genuinely curious about their medical school patients into efficient providers who were courteous but remote from any understanding of their patients' lives. A review of the literature showed that this was now perceived as a national problem, and he set out to create a curriculum to reverse this trend.*

**Crump B. Professional Identity Curriculum at the University of Louisville Trover Campus: Reflection and Meaning in Medical Education. The Journal of the Kentucky Academy of Family Physicians. Winter 2017;88:18.**

As medical students and residents learn clinical medicine, they not only learn to act like their faculty (often termed professionalism), they actually become them, incorporating the physician role into how they see themselves. Something happens in this process where the curves of empathy begin to diverge even in college and medical school and this divergence accelerates during residency and practice. Learners who trend in an arc upward toward the "A" side look beyond impressing their faculty to get good evaluation scores and the focus on good test scores and begin to spend time with patients that doesn't show in their grade. Those trending in an arc downward toward the "B" side often see patient care as a means to the end of securing good grades, the "best" residency and fellowship, and the highest income and prestige. Like the Faustian bargain, those on the "B" side may end up cynical and burned out, with resulting addiction, depression, divorce, and ill health.

The medical literature does not give many details to help us understand what happens during this professional identity formation process, but it is becoming clear that reflective exercises along the way help learners find their "A" side. These reflective exercises can be creative writing, career eulogies, drawing (even as simply as a "comic" with text balloons above stick figures), music, art, and non-medical literature appreciation. In fact, any exercise that causes the learner to pause, reflect, and find meaning in everyday activities seems to be effective. We began a formal curriculum in 2015 including baseline and subsequent measures of empathy with our students and residents as they experience various reflective exercises and have learned from their feedback. Our hope is that we can give each learner a "nudge" towards the "A" side. Some of the results of these exercises are included in our journal, and we urge you to try them yourself during that rare moment of quiet reflection, and then find a trusted colleague and share.

**Crump WJ, Ziegler CH, Fricker RS. A residency professional identity curriculum and a longitudinal measure of empathy in a community-based program. Journal of Regional Medical Campuses. 2018:1(4).**

## ABSTRACT
*Background*

Empathy as an attribute of physicians is considered desirable, and most studies have shown a progressive decline of measured empathy during residency training. Development of a professional identity during residency is also considered desirable. To study this process, empathy measures were used before and after implementation of a structured professional identity curriculum to determine the effect of the curriculum on empathy among a group of family medicine residents.

## METHODS

The Jefferson Scale of Empathy was completed by 18 residents at all three years of training before, immediately after a six month professional identity curriculum intervention, and six months after the curriculum was completed. The curriculum included one hour luncheon sessions on concepts of profession, burnout, and cynicism as well as thoughtful use of electronic medical records, prevention and management of burnout, mindfulness techniques and reflective writing and drawing.

## RESULTS

Similar to previous publications, a decline in empathy across the academic year was found, with a significant decline six months after the end of the curriculum. Residents who attended more professional identity sessions showed a non-significant smaller decline, and there were large standard deviations among each training level with some individual residents showing little change across the year. Evaluations of the curriculum were largely positive.

## CONCLUSIONS

This professional identity curriculum in this group of residents may have temporarily mitigated the decline in measured empathy that has been described among residents in other settings. Results support some aspects of empathy as a trait in some residents rather than a state that is amenable to a training effect. Alternatively, some residents show little change in high empathy scores across time, suggesting resilience despite the stress of training. Further study in this residency including longitudinal empathy measurements, individual resident's preference for strategies for burnout prevention and the association with changes in empathy, and focus groups is ongoing. Other programs' experience with these issues is needed to add to sample size and diversity of training environments to discern which changes are significant and generalizable.

## INTRODUCTION

Empathy is often listed as a desirable attribute for physicians, but attempts to define it are challenging, and measuring it is even more difficult. The developers of the Jefferson Scale of Empathy assign the more emotional aspects to the concept of sympathy, while empathy is more cognitive and includes an inquisitiveness to understand the other's feelings without completely joining with them or feeling the full depth of their emotion. In this view, empathy is something that can be developed but requires significant effort, and is more accurate and less affected by the physician's own emotional state. Oversimplified, empathy is "I understand your suffering," while sympathy is "I feel your pain." Several publications have shown a significant decline in empathy during the clinical years of medical school and a small decline across all years of residency training.

Professional identity is also an important concept in understanding the process of medical education. Professionalism is a code of behavior that physicians in training can learn and follow without internalizing. Professional identity is the state of actually becoming a physician when the values of the profession are internalized. At the final stage of identity development, the self is defined by thinking, feeling, and acting like a physician. This process is complex, and is dependent on one's pre-existing identity, socialization including availability of role models, and symbols and rituals. The working definitions used during the development of our professional identity curriculum were that professionalism is what you do when someone is watching, and professional identity is who you are.

There is current interest in studying the experience of medical trainees as they develop identities and learn empathy. Reflective exercises such as composing narratives, participation in organized study of art, film, music and literature, and opportunities to learn and practice mindfulness have been used to facilitate this development.

Efforts directed specifically to enhance empathy have included those for medical students[9] and residents in training. The general trend regardless of the instrument used was that measured scores increased after the intervention, and some have shown that the change was sustained for at least 10 weeks.

Our intent with this project was to determine the change in empathy among a group of family medicine residents as they were exposed to a structured professional identity (PI) curriculum. Our hypothesis was that the expected decrease in empathy during an academic year would be moderated by the PI curriculum and that the more sessions a resident attended, the larger would be the effect.

## METHOD

The three year family medicine residency is a community-based program with 6 residents at each level, unopposed, established in the mid-1970s, and is set in a town of 20,000 in western Kentucky. All 18 residents participated in this project during academic year 2015-2016. The host hospital and outpatient facilities were established in the 1950s as an early rural integrated health system, and have also supported a regional medical school clinical campus since 1998. The hospital has 80 physicians representing most specialties of secondary care, but also provides cardiac bypass procedures and a regional cancer center, serving as a referral site for portions of 5 surrounding counties.

As part of a regular lunchtime residency conference series, the first author, who is the dean of the regional medical school campus, provided six monthly 45 minute sessions as the basis for the professional identity (PI) curriculum during the 2015-2016 academic year. A family physician, he serves as the primary faculty for the residency in obstetrics and teaches occasionally in both the residency clinic and on the general adult medicine hospital teaching service, and staffs most resident deliveries. These sessions were interspersed with more typical sessions taught by him that were focused on obstetrics topics and actual case reviews of resident patients. The curriculum is shown in Table 1. The conference series is required for all residents on in-town rotations barring true emergencies or documented illness. Residents do have inpatient pediatric and dermatology rotations out of town, and occasionally the inpatient service in town is so busy that the senior resident and intern on service are not able to attend noon conference. Attendance was recorded by a senior resident for each session.

## A PROFESSIONAL IDENTITY CURRICULUM

*Session — Component*

1. Definitions

    - A profession is a social role characterized by having special knowledge and not just special skills, pursued largely for the good of others, and its value is not measured only by financial return

    - Burnout is a mismatch between what you thought you'd be doing and what you're actually doing, often associated with disengagement, fatigue, and physical symptoms

    - A cynic is someone who cannot imagine that anyone's behavior is motivated by anything but self-interest

    - Cynicism rises and empathy falls across training time. Group discussion of potential causes

2. The i-patient

    - The i-patient is the digital representation in an electronic record that "becomes" the patient

    - Discussions of articles on the i-patient

    - Why so much effort spent keeping the i-patient healthy? (meaningful use certification, billing, liability)

    - Strategies for keeping the i-patient healthy while making time for connecting with the real patient (empowering medical assistants to document, use of scribes, and standing orders for simple issues)

    - Strategies for breaking learned helplessness as a resident

3. Preventing burnout — Strategies reported by long-time practitioners

- Make choices congruent with your values
- Make time for friends and family, avoid the "god complex"
- Practice some religious or spiritual activity daily
- Pay attention to self-care (nutrition, exercise)
- Work to adopt a positive outlook, learn to re-frame
- Choose a job that gives you control over your workload
- Find meaning in daily work rather than hold out for vacations
- Find a mentor and stay in touch

4. Mindfulness Techniques
   - "Career Eulogy" reflective writing
   - "Mindfulness is the opposite of multitasking"
   - Self-awareness including breathing and tension awareness
   - Cultivate a curiosity of the unknown
   - Practice being completely present- the doorknob pause

5. Managing current burnout
   - Recognize your tendencies
   - Workaholic- responds to challenges by doing more of the same
   - Superhero- every problem is theirs to solve
   - Perfectionist- standard is no mistakes, and expects the same from everyone around them
   - Lone ranger- works best alone, and micromanages tasks that could be delegated
   - The energy account (doctors keep working even when their batteries run down, so learn how to re-charge)
   - Physical energy account (rest, exercise, nutrition)
   - Emotional energy account (invest in healthy relationships)

- Spiritual energy account (connect with your personal sense of purpose)

6. Group reflective exercise

    - Provided with a template, draw a "comic" with stick figures and text balloons
    - Your best experience with patients in the last 6 months
    - Your worst experience with patients in the last 6 months
    - Share what you drew and reflect on what you learned

At the beginning of the first session of the academic year, the Jefferson Scale of Empathy (JSE) was completed by all attendees. Each form had the resident's name included for later matching, but a senior resident placed each into an envelope confidentially, and participants were assured that a research assistant unknown to them would place an ID number and subsequently no one would be able to connect their responses to their name. A residency staff member then had each resident who missed this conference complete the survey within 3 days, again with confidentiality preserved. Anonymous curriculum evaluations were completed after the fifth session. The JSE was completed again after all 6 PI sessions were completed and no sessions were held in the second half of the academic year. The JSE was then completed again at the end of the academic year, approximately 6 months after the last PI session. The Baptist Health Madis

IBM SPSS Statistics for Windows (version 24.0, 2016, IBM Corporation, Armonk, NY, 877-426-6006) was used to analyze the data. Between groups repeated measures analysis of variance methods were used to analyze the JSE data across the academic year time points and between number of sessions attended (coded into two groups) and academic year of residents. Statistical significance was set by convention at $p < 0.05$.

# RESULTS

All absences from PI sessions were excused absences because of verified illness, clinical responsibilities, or out of town rotations. Among all 18 residents, 1 resident attended all 6 sessions, 7 attended 5, 4 attended 4, 4 attended 3, and 2 attended 2 sessions. The anonymous evaluations were largely positive. Comparing differences of means, there were no significant differences comparing PG-1 to PG-2 to PG-3 at any of the time points. Across the academic year, there were no significant changes in the means in the PG-1 and PG-2 classes. In the PG-3 class, there was a significant decline in JSE scores from baseline (Mean=117.50) to completion of the PI curriculum (Mean=109.17, p=0.037) as well as baseline to 6 months after the conclusion of the PI curriculum (Mean=105.50, p=0.029).

The decrement in empathy scores was variable after the PI curriculum based on how many of the 6 sessions the individual resident attended, but none were statistically significant. Residents who only attended 3 or fewer sessions decreased by a mean of 6.83 points while residents who attended 5 or more decreased only by a mean 0.38 points. Residents who attended 4 or fewer sessions decreased an intermediate degree, by a mean of 4.50 points.

## DISCUSSION

The professional identity curriculum was well received by these residents, and may have partially mitigated the decrease in empathy measured by the JSE that accelerated in the second half of the year. We did not use a measure of professional identity itself, and it is possible that our sessions facilitated that development. Our findings highlight the issue of whether empathy is a trait that doesn't change much (inborn, or developed at a very young age) or truly a state (as supported by the developers of the JSE) that could be strengthened as a physician's identity coalesces. Of the few previous reports using the JSE among residents, a cross-sectional study measuring JSE scores showed a non-significant downward trend across the three years in an internal medicine residency, but there were no longitudinal surveys to show how individual residents changed over time. In studies of medical students, JSE scores in the M-3 year correlated to ratings of empathy by residency program directors three years later, but this could again support that empathy is a trait with little change over time. Longitudinal studies in one medical school did show a decrease during the M-3 year when compared with measures done in the M-2 year.

With such large standard deviations and marked individual changes, inferential statistics for differences of means may not give the best view of empathy among groups of residents. Supporting our prediction that the PI curriculum would have a positive effect on empathy was the "dose effect" of the number of sessions attended showing a differential more positive JSE score, but again the difference of means was not significant. This may be simply a problem with small sample size or the fact that means hide the important individual variability. Empathy for some residents may be predominantly a trait that will be changed little by a curriculum and for others it may be more of a state that is changed both by their everyday experiences and curriculum.

One PG-1 showed a large drop in JSE in the first half of the year despite attending 3 PI sessions, and recovered somewhat. One PG-2 showed a large drop in the second half of the year, after attending 5 PI sessions. Conversely, it appears that some residents are resistant to the expected decline in measured empathy during training. Further detailed analysis of these residents' attitudes and experiences prior to and during residency merit further study. The two reflective exercises in the PI sessions were collected and recorded by ID number, and further studies of their content may also provide insight into how these residents differ from the mean.

## LIMITATIONS

Generalization of our findings must be limited to similar residents in similar environments. The effects of having a faculty member facilitate the "softer" PI elements who is also recognized as an experienced clinician in the hospital and clinic may make a difference in both acceptability and effectiveness. With our findings of clear trends in means without statistical significance, small group size may be an issue. Other programs can add to our understanding by replicating our efforts with similar measures.

Already mentioned is the possibility that using group means may obscure important individual differences in such a non-quantitative concept as empathy. The JSE is well validated, but it may not measure exactly what is intended. We have group focus sessions scheduled where we will ask participants to predict what changes should be seen at all three levels of postgraduate training, share with them what we found, and then listen to their interpretations of their meaning.

As with any educational intervention that is not randomized, there is a possibility of systemic bias, where residents who are predisposed to be affected by the topic choose to attend, or vice versa. The lack of a true control group is an important limitation, but the number of sessions attended is as close to randomly assigned as possible in this environment. The sessions were deliberately held on different days of the week at different points in the month, and there was no systemic pattern for which residents were assigned to out of town rotations or otherwise were unable to attend, and attendance was mandatory. We do not have historical controls in the year before the PI curriculum was begun, but in subsequent years the PI curriculum was diluted and spread across an entire year, and we continue to measure the JSE at the beginning of each academic year.

## FURTHER RESEARCH NEEDED

Use of the JSE in other residency programs along with published details of their PI curriculum would be helpful. In our program we will use focus groups to understand the process better as well as to design studies to describe more carefully the residents who appear to be resistant to the expected decline in measures of empathy as training proceeds.

# DEVELOPING A PROFESSIONAL IDENTITY CURRICULUM, CONT.

*The longitudinal design used to collect individual paired results on empathy and burnout measures was unique in the medical literature, and this allowed Dr. Crump's group to make an important contribution. While many publications had demonstrated the decline in empathy and rise in burnout during residency training, these studies used a cross sectional design and so could not answer the question of which came first. One school of thought held that if doctors began to feel too much empathy for their suffering patients, burnout would follow. The other theory was that everyday frustrations and loss of autonomy caused burnout to rise first and then empathy would decline. In the key publication below, Dr. Crump's group showed that in their residents, burnout clearly rose first, followed by a decline in empathy.*

Crump WJ, Ziegler C, Fricker S. Empathy and Burnout During Residency: Which Changes First? Fam Med. 2022;54(8):640-643. Copyright 2022, Society of Teachers of Family Medicine. Used by permission.

## ABSTRACT

### Background and Objectives

The issue of declining empathy and increasing burnout among residents is of concern for most programs. Numerous studies have shown these changes in both medical students and residents. However, the sequence of empathy decline and increasing burnout is unresolved and most studies have been cross-sectional. This paper reports an individually paired longitudinal analysis intended to clarify the sequence of these changes.

## METHODS

Beginning in 2017, 34 Family Medicine residents across all 3 years of training at a rural program completed an established empathy survey and a previously validated single burnout question at the start of each year and at the mid-point. First, the empathy score for each resident was aligned with the next following burnout measure and then the reverse sequence with burnout aligned with the following empathy score were analyzed.

## RESULTS

With 125 responses to 133 survey opportunities we saw a 94% response rate. Empathy scores across residency years decreased slightly and then improved almost to baseline. However, the ANOVA test for quadratic trend was not significant. The burnout measure increased significantly over the residency years (J-T Statistic = 4.89, $p < 0.001$). The correlation of the empathy score changing first showed a nonsignificant correlation ($R_s=-.150$, $p=0.133$). The Spearman's Rho of the burnout measure changing first was significant ( $R_s=-.300$, $p=0.006$).

## CONCLUSIONS

In this group of residents, changes in burnout occurred before changes in empathy. If further research supports this finding, residency programs could focus more on efforts to address burnout to mitigate decreases in empathy.

## INTRODUCTION

Most studies show a decline in measured empathy across the clinical years of medical school as well as residency.[1-3] Burnout is generally characterized by depersonalization, emotional exhaustion, and loss of a sense of personal accomplishment, all leading to a rise in cynicism.[4] The primary source of burnout in residency is seen as stemming from high job demands in the setting of low individual autonomy.[5-7] The sequence of these changes is an unresolved issue. Some believe that physicians who connect too strongly with their patients might actually suffer worse burnout.4 The opposing view is that since empathy is viewed as protective against burnout, empathy must decrease before burnout increases.8

The most comprehensive review comparing empathy and burnout in medical professionals showed a negative relationship.9 The authors point out that all previous studies have been cross-sectional, and without a sequenced paired longitudinal study, the issue of which comes first could not be addressed.9,10 The present study was designed to address this question of sequence.

## METHODS

Our residency, begun in 1971, is located in a town of 20,000 in a rural area in the upper southeast, with six residents in each year, with no other residencies in town.11 The site is also host for our regional rural medical school campus, with the main campus in a metropolitan community 160 miles away.12

Beginning in 2016, 49 residents completed the empathy survey (see Table 1)13 on paper during a regular administrative meeting just as the academic year began or ended, and at the mid-point of the academic year. A single burnout question was added to the back of the page in December 2017 that asked 34 residents to choose one of 5 statements reporting increasing burnout (see Figure 1).14 We used the single-item burnout measure rather than the full Maslach Inventory to increase completion rate that has been reported to be a problem with the longer survey.9 Each survey was matched by individual resident. If a resident completed at least one full year (2 surveys) during the study period, regardless of training year, their data was included. Two resident empathy and burnout responses were excluded from the analysis for not following directions. The host hospital IRB designated the project as exempt.

First, for the empathy measure, analysis of variance was used where a polynomial test of quadratic trend was performed. For the burnout question, a Jonckheere-Terpstra Test of linear trend was performed. Next, the empathy score for each resident was aligned with the next following burnout measure. For example, a resident's baseline empathy score was aligned with their mid-year PGY 1 burnout measure and a resident's mid-year empathy PGY 1 score was aligned with their post PGY 1 burnout measure, and so on. If significant, this would support that the empathy score changed first. A similar alignment was created where the resident's burnout measure was aligned with the next following empathy score. If significant, this would support that the burnout measure changed first. After the alignment, a Spearman's Rho was performed correlating empathy score with the following burnout measure, and correlating burnout measure with the following empathy score. Significance was set at p<0.05 and all tests were 2-tailed. SPSS version 27.0 was used for statistical analysis. Figures were created with the R package GGPLOT.15

## RESULTS

Of 133 opportunities to complete a survey, 125 responses were usable for a response rate of 94%. Demographics are shown in Table 2. The empathy scores across the three residency years decreased slightly and then improved somewhat back to baseline. The ANOVA test of quadratic trend was not significant. Burnout measure increased significantly over residency years, J-T Statistic = 4.89, p < 0.001. (See Table 3 and Figure 1.) The correlation of the empathy score changing first showed a nonsignificant correlation, Rs=-.150 (95% CIs=-.33, .05), p=0.133. The Spearman's Rho of burnout measure changing first was significant, Rs=-.300, (95% CIs=-.49, -.09), p=0.006.

## DISCUSSION

Our longitudinal results clearly show that in our residents, burnout increases prior to any decrease in empathy. While methods to maintain empathy including reflective exercises such as composing narratives, participation in organized study of art, film, music and literature, and opportunities to learn and practice mindfulness may be useful,16 scarce residency resources and time may be better spent to address causes of burnout in the individual program. Focus groups with our residents prior to some recent program improvements showed that adequate sleep and minimizing administrative work unassociated with learning were ranked as most important overall and first year residents were concerned with learning a new electronic medical record and adapting to a new city.17

A recent national study of 2509 Family Medicine residents showed that although burnout scores were not associated with in-training exam scores, they were correlated with failure to meet the professional conduct and accountability milestone. This study also reported that adequate salary given local cost of living is important.18 If our goal is to produce empathetic professionals, attention to local causes of burnout seems wise.

## *Limitations and Strengths*

As with almost all previous reports on resident empathy and burnout, selection bias and limited generalizability are a concern with reports from a single site. Our findings should be generalized only to similar sites and similar residents. By using a standing meeting for survey administration, we got a 94% response rate compared to previous studies that had response rates of 35% to 80%.

Surveys produce quantifiable results, but with concepts as nebulous as empathy and burnout, focus groups are important. We have reported some results from this residency previously, and we will continue those efforts.17 We also invite other programs to replicate our studies and combine results across programs.

## CONCLUSIONS

In our residents, changes in burnout occur prior to changes in empathy. If similar findings are reported in other sites, strengthened efforts to address program-specific sources of burnout may mitigate the decrease in empathy seen in some residents during training.

## *References*

1. Hojat M, Vergare MJ, Maxwell K, et al. The devil is in the third year: a longitudinal study of erosion of empathy in medical school. Acad Med. 2009;84(9):1182-91. doi:10.1097/ACM.0b013e3181b17e55

2. Bellini LM, Shea JA. Mood change and empathy decline persist during three years of internal medicine training. Acad Med. 2005;80(2):164-7. doi:10.1097/00001888-200502000-00013

3. Rosen IM, Gimotty PA, Shea JA, Bellini LM. Evolution of sleep quantity, sleep deprivation, mood disturbances, empathy, and burnout among interns. Acad Med. 2006;81(1):82-5. doi:10.1097/00001888-200601000-00020

4. Maslach C, Jackson SE. The measurement of experienced burnout. Journal of Organizational Behavior. 1981;2(2):99-113. doi:10.1002/job.4030020205

5. Thomas NK. Resident burnout. JAMA. 2004;292(23):2880-9. doi:10.1001/jama.292.23.2880

6. Buck K, Williamson M, Ogbeide S, Norberg B. Family Physician Burnout and Resilience: A Cross-Sectional Analysis. Fam Med. 2019;51(8):657-63. doi:10.22454/FamMed.2019.424025

7. Lebensohn P, Dodds S, Benn R, et al. Resident wellness behaviors: relationship to stress, depression, and burnout. Fam Med. 2013;45(8):541-9.

8. Zenasni F, Boujut E, Woerner A, Sultan S. Burnout and empathy in primary care: three hypotheses. Br J Gen Pract. 2012;62(600):346-7. doi:10.3399/bjgp12X652193

9. Wilkinson H, Whittington R, Perry L, Eames C. Examining the relationship between burnout and empathy in healthcare professionals: A systematic review. Burn Res. 2017;6:18-29. doi:10.1016/j.burn.2017.06.003

10. Thirioux B, Birault F, Jaafari N. Empathy Is a Protective Factor of Burnout in Physicians: New Neuro-Phenomenological Hypotheses Regarding Empathy and Sympathy in Care Relationship. Front Psychol. 2016;7:763. doi:10.3389/fpsyg.2016.00763

11. Martin D. A Short History of Trover Clinic with Commentary. McClanahan Publishing House; 1989.

12. Crump WJ, Fricker RS, Ziegler CH, Wiegman DL. Increasing the Rural Physician Workforce: A Potential Role for Small Rural Medical School Campuses. J Rural Health. 2016;32(3):254-9. doi:10.1111/jrh.12156

13. Hojat M, Gonnella JS. Eleven Years of Data on the Jefferson Scale of Empathy-Medical Student Version (JSE-S): Proxy Norm Data and Tentative Cutoff Scores. Med Princ Pract. 2015;24(4):344-50. doi:10.1159/000381954

14. Rohland BM, Kruse GR, Rohrer JE. Validation of a single-item measure of burnout against the Maslach Burnout Inventory among physicians. Stress and Health. 2004;20(2):75-9. doi:10.1002/smi.1002

15. Wickham H. Elegant Graphics for Data Analysis Ggplot Website. Accessed February 3, 2021. https://ggplot2.tidyverse.org

16. Hojat M. Ten approaches for enhancing empathy in health and human services cultures. J Health Hum Serv Adm. 2009;31(4):412-50.

17. Crump W, Ziegler C, Fricker R. Does empathy really decline during residency training? A longitudinal look at changes in measured empathy in a community program. J Regional Medical Campuses 2021. Accepted for publication

18. Davis C, Krishnasamy M, Morgan ZJ, Bazemore AW, Peterson LE. Academic Achievement, Professionalism, and Burnout in Family Medicine Residents. Fam Med. 2021 Jun;53(6):423-432. doi:10.22454/FamMed.2021.541354.

## ACKNOWLEDGEMENTS

We would like to recognize Debbie Peake, staff support in our residency, for her assistance in getting surveys completed on time.

Table 1. Examples of three questions used in the Jefferson Scale of Empathy (a)

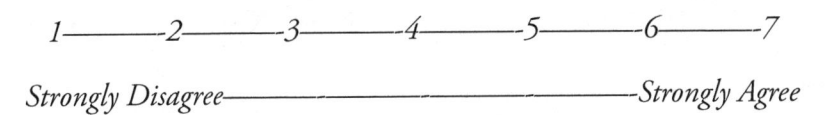

*1———2———3———4———5———6———7*

*Strongly Disagree————————————————Strongly Agree*

12b. Asking patients about what is happening in their personal lives is not helpful in understanding their physical complaints.

14b. I believe that emotion has no place in the treatment of medical illness.

20. I believe that empathy is an important therapeutic factor in medical treatment.

a. The JSE has 20 items, each ranked on a Likert scale from 1 to 7, with higher scores representing more measured empathy. It has reversed items that are accounted for in the total scoring. Subscales are not reported, and it has a normal distribution.13

b. The scores for these questions are reversed when calculating the JSE total score.

Figure 1. Mean results of resident responses to single item burnout measure by time of survey

The Jonckheere-Terpstra Test of Linear Trend for the Single Item Burnout Measure was significant, $p<0.001$.

Residents were asked to choose one of 5 statements (14):

1. I enjoy my work. I have no symptoms of burnout;
2. Occasionally I am under stress, and I don't always have as much energy as I once did, but I don't feel burned out;
3. I am definitely burning out and have one or more symptoms of burnout, such as physical and emotional exhaustion;
4. The symptoms of burnout that I'm experiencing won't go away. I think about frustration at work a lot;
5. I feel completely burned out and often wonder if I can go on. I am at the point where I may need some changes or may need to seek some sort of help

Table 3: Mean, Standard Deviation, and 95% Confidence Limits of Jefferson Scale of Empathy and Single Item Burnout Measure

Mean (SD), [95.0% Confidence Limits]

| | |
|---|---|
| Empathy Scale Baseline (N=29) | 111.4 (14.0) [106.1, 116.7] |
| Mid PGY-1 (N=29) | 108.2 (19.1) [100.9, 115.4] |
| Post PGY-1 (N=27) | 104.4 (14.7) [98.6, 110.2] |
| Mid PGY-2 (N=25) | 105.4 (16.8) [98.5, 112.3] |
| Post PGY-2 (N=27) | 106.4 (16.0) [100.1, 112.8] |
| Mid PGY-3 (N=27) | 104.7 (15.3) [98.6, 110.7] |
| Post PGY-3 (N=28) | 107.4 (16.1) [101.1, 113.6] |
| | |
| Single Item Burnout Measure Baseline (N=13) | 1.23 (0.44) [0.97, 1.50] |
| Mid PGY-1 (N=22) | 1.68 (0.89) [1.29, 2.08] |
| Post PGY-1 (N=14) | 2.14 (1.03) [1.55, 2.74] |
| Mid PGY-2 (N=20) | 2.30 (0.86) [1.90, 2.70] |
| Post PGY-2 (N=14) | 2.36 (0.93) [1.82, 2.89] |
| Mid PGY-3 (N=21) | 2.62 (1.16) [2.09, 3.15] |
| Post PGY-3 (N=16) | 2.62 (0.96) [2.11, 3.14] |

# JOURNAL EDITORIAL BOARDS: TIME TO THINK AND WRITE, 2005-2017

*While continuing to build the Trover Campus and later to modify the professional identity curriculum and publishing 8 articles covering lessons learned, opportunities to reflect and write essays found Dr. Crump. He was asked to take over as editor of the state academy family medicine journal and serve as an officer, ultimately leading to the presidency in 2006. He was also invited to join the state medical association journal editorial board. In these roles he was expected to contribute an essay to each journal roughly quarterly. This provided a welcome respite from the day-to-day work, and an opportunity to reflect on the important issues of the day from his perspective, a spot he sometimes referred to as the "crow's nest." This ushered in a remarkable 12 year period of productivity that is included in its entirety below. Of these essays, Dr. Crump says that since in medicine what was old always becomes new again, the musings may be helpful to future physicians.*

### From your president: Who's not here?

As I stood to take the oath of office at our May meeting, I was first focused on repeating the words that Larry Fields guided me through. It was especially meaningful to have Larry, the President-elect of our national Academy, conducting this ceremony. Then as I gained confidence that my ability to repeat lofty words truly hadn't left me, I began to look around the room and consider who wasn't there.

First, of course, my 90 year-old father. He's as mentally sharp as ever, but the trip from Savannah would have been too much for him. My mother, the perfect grandmother, who was taken from us far too soon - too soon for my children to really know this remarkable woman. My three sisters and their husbands weren't there- only because I didn't ask them to make the drive. I know they would have, because that's what families do. My oldest daughter and my son and their families couldn't make it, but my other two daughters and a fiancé did. And my wife Vanessa, who has put up with me for almost 25 years, was there for me as always.

Then I began to think of all the students who I know are now Family Medicine residents in our state, and all the young family docs who are just beginning their life's work. I wondered if they even knew about all the changes in their Academy: that one of our own was stepping up onto the national stage with a clear message on the value of what we do; that our state chapter has a new Executive who has breathed new life into our efforts; that their colleagues with maybe only a few years left of active practice were here dedicating themselves to learning about electronic health records - because that's what family doctors do - we do what we need to do to get the best for our patients.

For those who could not make it to the meeting, let me assure you that these are exciting times. I have been fortunate to have been associated with the Alabama AFP for 12 years, the Texas chapter for 6, and now our own for 7 years. The energy and commitment I have sensed over the last year as we crafted a new strategic plan and set about getting it done is as strong as I have seen in any chapter at any time.

We redesigned our committee structure to be lean and effective. About the time I finish writing this piece, I will join in the first of a series of teleconferences with the co-chairs of these new groups. If you care about the future of our specialty, these folks can use your energy - choose a committee and let Gerry Stover know. One of the most remarkable initiatives grew from the new leadership committee, comprised of the former chapter presidents. They have pledged to make a personal visit to the practice of every family doctor newly setting up practice in Kentucky over the next year. The message will be clear: you're welcome here and we need you in your Academy.

Over the next year I will visit with each medical school Family Medicine interest group and FM residency in our Commonwealth. My message will be on the definition of success. As I have rediscovered my own faith recently, I have had occasion to reflect on just what being a servant means. The feeling we have when we hear someone say "hey, that's my doctor," or the sense of privilege to be the guide to births and deaths in the families' lives that we share- this is what it's all about. To paraphrase a bit, a plaque that my daughter gave me several years ago sums it up: Some measure success by the size of their house or the net worth of their stock portfolio. The real measure of success is one you cannot spend. It's the way your patients describe you when talking to a friend.

I feel that I am blessed to have the best job in the world, and I'm going to share that message with anyone who will listen. This I do solemnly swear.

## WELCOME TO OUR NEW EDITOR

We are pleased to welcome Dr. Bill Crump as the Editor of our Academy's journal. Dr. Crump is the Associate Dean of the U of L Trover Campus in Madisonville, and continues an active practice including obstetrics. He was editor-in-chief of the Life Support and Biosphere Science Journal when he worked with the NASA as medical monitor for Space Station design, and was on the editorial board of the Texas Journal of Rural Health. He currently serves on the editorial board of Family Practice Recertification, and has authored more than 130 publications. Concerning his new role, Dr. Crump says; "I am very aware of the passion and commitment that Dr. Zukoff had for this publication for almost 20 years. I hope to highlight the tradition of this great Academy while bringing our readers word of issues that affect their daily lives and renew their spirit."

Dr. Crump invites ideas for articles, especially stories about family docs who have made a difference in their communities. He also invites Academy members who would like to be feature editors for columns such as news from our residencies, stories from the trenches, and a word from your future colleagues (students and residents). Similarly, nominations of lay people who could contribute to a feature called "what your patients are hearing about FP" would also be welcome.

# FROM THE EDITOR
## October 2005

Much is changing with your Journal. I pledge to keep some of the tradition alive while bringing you current events and issues. I am truly pleased to introduce our new Associate Editors, Charles Kodner in Louisville and Steve Wrightson in Lexington. Twice a year, each will take the lead in producing an issue. We hope to include brief clinical studies and timely topic reviews brought to you from a uniquely Family Medicine viewpoint. We also want to share the stories of family doctors throughout the Commonwealth that paint a picture of who are and what we do.

Borrowing a term from the Future of Family Medicine Report, we believe each Kentuckian deserves a medical home. This home should be tended by that person's family doctor that may not actually provide each and every service needed, but who manages the "basket of services." When a patient needs a service not provided by his doctor, a consultant is chosen carefully based on the unique knowledge of the totality of that patient as an individual. We all have stories of how knowing someone as a person has affected health choices and outcomes. We ask you to share your stories with us, maybe answering the question: "Why in the world would this patient do that?"

I'll start with one of my own. Returning from a week away from practice, a young woman who I had seen for 6-8 visits over about a year appeared on my schedule again. Entering the room, I could see she was distraught. Holding a sheet of paper in her hand, she looked up and said, "I'm so glad you're back!" It took the next ten minutes to recreate the 2 visits to the urgent care center, 1 ED visit, a cardiology consult, and a treadmill test that had transpired as I was at CME. It started with just heart racing and "feeling funny." The nurse practitioner at the urgent care center said the EKG didn't look just right, and suggested a cardiologist visit (worry begins). Then it turned out that the first appointment was 3 weeks away (more worry).

Then a brief episode of chest pain and shortness of breath resulted in another urgent care visit 2 days later, where she was sent straight to the ED. The ED folks seemed to the patient to be really worried, and before she knew it she had an IV in her arm and some bitter TNG spray in her mouth that only gave her a headache. The ED doctor said the EKG looked fine to him, but scheduled a treadmill in the AM (even more worry). The treadmill wiped her out, and the doctor said it was inconclusive and scheduled a cardiac cath. The paper in her hand described the instructions for this test, scheduled for tomorrow. She was now really worried. "What should I do?" she said.

All of this made sense to me. I had seen her twice with fleeting symptoms with normal findings before I asked if she had any insight into why she is so sensitive to such feelings. Through some tears, she explained that her father had been killed in a mining accident when she was in fourth grade, and she had been worried about her own death ever since. Now she was married, had a 7 year-old daughter, and every little health issue loomed like it could be her last. After that, she would come in with a small reactive lymph node convinced she had leukemia or a rash that she thought was spotted fever. Each time I would carefully examine her and order basic lab as indicated. When I went back in the room with the results, ready for a difficult time reassuring her, each time it was easier. We had finally gotten to the point where she would say "All I need to hear is that it's okay- if you say so."

I also knew that her husband left on a week-long business trip about the time her last round of symptoms began. I reviewed her low-risk history, again examined her, and repeated a normal EKG. I was all prepared to talk about predictive value and false positive treadmill tests, when she said:" Just tell me what you would tell your daughter in this situation." I could honestly say that I wouldn't recommend the cath. Hearing that her husband would be back tomorrow, we were both okay with waiting, with a dose of hydroxyzine tonight at bedtime.

Although this visit just got coded as a 91214, it was important. If I had not known her well enough, I could have easily said to proceed with the cath. I could have let my own slight uneasiness show, making hers worse. Instead, I played the role of her doctor, tending her medical home. Since then I have delivered her second child and seen her husband through a couple of minor illnesses (that she thought were life-threatening). Family doctoring is just so much more than CPT codes and making referrals.

I invite you to comment on my story or share your own. Call or Email whichever Associate Editor is closest to you, and he will help you get it ready for publication. The family doctor's story is just too good not to be shared.

**Crump WJ. How bright our future? Journal of the Kentucky Academy of Family Physicians. 2006; 54: 1-3.**

As I accepted the role of your president at our May meeting, I pledged to visit each residency program and medical school in our state. The purpose was to bring a positive message about the future of our discipline and to learn more about the opportunities and concerns at each site.

I completed those visits last fall, and it was truly energizing. I re-learned how wide our state is and again learned that there is no substitute for a personal visit. When this process was discussed at our last Board meeting, it was agreed that these visits should become part of the tradition of the presidential year for the KAFP. I gave a short address at each site, focusing on the definition of success. I first asked the group to provide some words describing a successful individual. With various degrees of prompting needed, the responses were remarkably similar at all sites. Under the category of "productivity," the words included the markers of financial independence: cars, houses, boats, designer clothes, horses, land, and (among the most cynical comment heard) trophy spouse. I then asked the participants to imagine the happiest physician they had known, and under the category of "meaning," I heard words like fulfilled, patient, compassionate, enthusiastic, satisfied, humble, fun-loving, and caring. The non-verbal change while making the second list was interesting. The hesitant revelation of cynical thoughts was replaced by a torrent of positive attributes and smiling faces. This interchange gives me renewed optimism for our future.

## PRODUCTIVITY

Next we spent some time talking about ways to ensure our future productivity. Using the Future of Family Medicine project as a backdrop and my personal experiences in practice in Alabama and Texas as examples, we constructed an image of the future of our practices. I painted the picture that includes a medical home for every American, tended by a caring family doctor. That doctor will be paid (not reimbursed) to do what we do best: manage the care of our patients. This includes the cognitive and procedural things we do ourselves, but it also includes payment for coordinating the basket of services needed by our patients. This image of the future also includes open access, with patients knowing that they can be seen the same day they call when really needed. I described a Medicaid managed care program that I worked with in Texas that used this model to decrease emergency room care significantly while paying a monthly management fee to us.

Then we discussed the shift to population-based practice that is in our future. I foresee that each family doctor will have a clear view of the needs of the 2000 or so souls that comprise her patient panel. Whether they enter the door of our practice in any given year, they are still our responsibility and our partners in promoting the health of the practice. I discussed my experience with an electronic medical record as clearly the best way to shift our focus to the population. How else can a doctor answer the questions: Are all the women in my practice getting mammograms at the correct time? Have all my hypertensives received dietary advice? Have all my diabetics been screened for proteinuria?-and countless others. With Pay for Performance on the horizon (see the last issue of our journal), I shared my experience with such a system. The lesson I learned is that physicians had better be at the table when the measures are chosen, and we'd better have a way to provide data that we trust.

Next I reminded the residents and students to commit to lifelong learning and keep an open mind to what services they will provide in the future, using my own experiences with maternity care and sports medicine as examples. Many in our culture change careers every 6-10 years, and the family doctor will almost surely change the focus of his work at least as often. We do what our patients need us to do, and change is the rule.

We closed this section by summarizing an article from one of our discipline's leaders that makes the case that the 15 minute visit model is obsolete. Group visits and virtual care are already here, and he makes a strong case for their future. I asked the participants to choose between two options. If you're a 55 year old with hypertension, option A is the traditional visit. This means leave work, drive to the doctor's office, find a place to park, pay your $25 co-pay, and wait in the waiting room. Then get your 6 minutes with your doctor, wait for your lab to be drawn, take your prescription to the pharmacy, wait some more, and get back to work and have to stay late to finish the day's tasks. Option B is to go to your personal, secure web site and leave a message for your doctor with your recent BP measurements. Later you get her response with advice, including electronic orders for lab to be drawn near your work at your convenience and a prescription sent to your pharmacy. For this you pay your $25 co-pay to your doctor's practice.

Once everyone was assured that face-to-face care was still available when needed and that good patient education is available, most chose option B, with the younger faces in the audience making the choice more enthusiastically. When one does the math, the doctor in this scenario can actually increase the number of patients cared for by 15-25% without an increase in staff by spreading out the frequency of required face-to-face visits. This model also allows for the longer personal visit needed in times of crisis. In a subscription or "retainer" style practice, wouldn't patients pay a monthly fee for this access at least equal to what they pay for Internet access or basic cell phone use? Time will tell.

## LEADERSHIP AND ADVOCACY

Next I made my case to the group that organized medicine needs them. To understand what the older docs bemoan as the loss of "the good old days," I suggested studying the "Taylorization" of modern medicine. In the 1900s, almost everything was made by skilled workers with knowledge handed down through generations using carefully protected trade secrets. The result was that the craftsmen set the style and pace of their work, and were well-rewarded. Frederick Winslow Taylor was a workshop supervisor at this time who set out to change the way work is accomplished. He broke complex tasks into small individual steps, analyzed each step, and devised the most efficient way to complete each. The outcome was nothing short of a revolution, applied to automobile construction by Henry Ford and fast food by Ray Kroc.

There were two results of this revolution. First, the increase in productivity provided the standard of living that characterizes developed nations even today. Second was the rise of a managerial class whose job it is to organize and supervise a highly regulated workplace. This is perhaps no better summarized than in a chilling quote from Taylor himself:

"In the past, man has been first. In the future, the system will be first."

This describes the crux of the challenge for the future of medicine in America. We physicians are trained as craftsmen and then enter practice where our activities are constrained by managers who do not understand our craft. Mind you, managers are not bad people – they just don't understand that everything that transpires between humans and their healers cannot be reduced to the most efficient set of steps that then can be measured precisely. So, do we curse the darkness or light a candle? I hear a lot of cursing in our doctors' lounge, but I choose to illuminate. Organized medicine is the best hope we have to maintain a group of physicians who understand the fallacy of the Taylorization of medicine. No one of us can carry the mantle of our guild every day, year in and year out, and still maintain a practice. So, we volunteer to take up this challenge for our elected year of service, or a few years on a key committee. What other real choice do we have?

Many physicians simply get worn-out by the long process of change in bureaucracy and politics – we're accustomed to seeing visible progress as we work. I used the example of liability reform in Texas with the group. When I practiced there in the mid 1990s, it was clear that real reform would only come when a group of key high court justices was replaced. Organized medicine in the state set about to make this happen, and the pace of the effort was almost imperceptible during the 6 years I was there. Last year, almost 10 years after the effort began, the laws were changed and withstood judicial review. The result is that hospital premiums that had increased 30% in 2003 dropped by 17% last year. Ten new insurance carriers entered the state, and there was a 70% drop in the number of lawsuits. No individual physician could claim this victory, but organized medicine in the state, comprised of hundreds of physicians who carried their load for their time, had made a difference. This was the basis of my plea to young physicians to become more involved in the KMA and KAFP. I hope some listened.

## FINDING MEANING

Having spent the first two-thirds of my talk on issues of productivity, we turned to focus on finding meaning in practice. Reflecting back on those words used to describe the happy physician, two groups of workers were described. The first toils through a burdensome job so that he can get to the next vacation or the ultimate prize, retirement. The second group seeks meaning in everyday work, finding fulfillment while earning a living. Several quotes from Dr. Rachel Remen's book formed the backdrop of this discussion (1). The first is as she describes the time just after the unexpected death of her medical partner. The office staff worked through their grief over the next few weeks, then noticed something unusual:

"Then the patients started coming. For almost a year afterwards, several times a week I would open the door to my office and find one of Hal's patients sitting in the common waiting room. At first I would worry that they didn't know about Hal and I would have to tell them, but they all knew. They had just come to the place where they had experienced his listening, his special way of seeing and valuing them, just to sit there for a bit, perhaps to think about difficult decisions which currently faced them. Many patients came. It was terribly, terribly moving."

At this point I asked the audience to consider whether they would like to be remembered in that way. Heads nodded, so I posed the question: Then what happens to us along the way? I shared my personal experience of working with idealistic, committed premed students who return to our summer programs after the first year of medical school as cynics, narrowly focused on the mechanics of medicine. I then watch the cynicism grow through medical school and peak late in residency. Fortunately, many rediscover their idealism late in residency or in the first few years of practice. Sadly, some do not. Dr. Remen provides a quote concerning her experience that says it well:

"In some ways, a medical training is like a disease. It would be years before I would fully recover from mine."

So I asked the group to consider how to speed this recovery – how can we find meaning even during medical school and residency? I proposed that one way is to fully experience the humanity of those we serve. Again, Dr. Remen provides a perspective:

"Sir William Osler, one of the fathers of modern medicine, is widely quoted as having said that objectivity is the essential quality of the true physician. What he actually said is different and more profound than that. The original quote was in Latin and it is the Latin word aequanimitas which is usually translated as "objectivity." But aequanimitas means "calmness of mind" or "inner peace." Inner peace is certainly the ultimate resource for those dealing with suffering on a daily basis. But this isn't something achieved by distancing yourself from the suffering around you. Inner peace is more a question of cultivating perspective, meaning, and wisdom even as life touches you with its pain. It is more a spiritual quality than a mental quality."

So, why the disconnect between work and meaning for so many physicians? Again, from Dr. Remen's book:

"Meaning may become a very practical matter for those of us who do difficult work or lead difficult lives. Meaning is strength. Physicians often seek their strength in competence. Indeed, competence and expertise are two of the most respected qualities in the medical subculture, as well as in our society. But important as they are, they are not sufficient to fully sustain us."

As physicians seek meaning in their work, too many become burned-out. Burnout has been described as the dislocation between what people are doing versus what they are expected to do. The result is often cynicism and multiple somatic symptoms. Asked to recall burned out physicians they've known, almost everyone in the audience nodded knowingly. Another phrase often used to describe burnout is "erosion of the soul."

I then shared some advice from one of my medical school mentors, Dr. Anderson Spickard. He and others reviewed the literature on physician renewal and burnout and published a review that summarized the successful strategies (2). We then reviewed the copies of the box I handed out, suggesting that they place it on their refrigerator at home or near where they dictate. I also invited the participants to keep in contact with me over the next year, letting me know which elements of this strategy were most useful to them.

I closed the talk expressing my wish for each of the participants to have a life full of meaning. A familiar story recounted in Dr. Remen's book emphasized the importance of finding meaning in everyday work:

"A great Italian psychiatrist, Roberto Assagioli, wrote a parable about interviewing three stonecutters building a cathedral in the fourteenth century. The effect of their sense of personal meaning on their experience of their work is the same as the effect meaning has for us today. When he asks the first stonecutter what he is doing, the man replies with bitterness that he is cutting stones into blocks, a foot by a foot by three quarters of a foot. With frustration, he describes a life in which he has done this over and over, and will continue to do it until he dies. The second stonecutter is also cutting stones into blocks, a foot by a foot by three quarters of a foot, but he replies in a somewhat different way. With warmth, he tells the interviewer that he is earning a living for his beloved family; through his work his children have clothes and food to grow strong, he and his wife have a home that they have filled with love. But it is the third man whose response gives us pause. In a joyous voice, he tells us of the privilege of participating in the building of this great cathedral, so strong that it will stand as a holy lighthouse for a thousand years."

"Competence may bring us satisfaction. Finding meaning in a familiar task often allows us to go beyond this and find in the most routine of tasks a deep sense of joy and even gratitude."

I see a bright future.

1. Remen RN. Kitchen table wisdom: Stories that heal. Riverhead Books. New York. 1996.
2. Spickard A, Gabbe SG, Christensen JF. Mid-career burnout in generalist and specialist physicians. JAMA 2002;288:1447-50.

Crump WJ. The Practice of Medicine: Ministry or Business? Journal of the Kentucky Academy of Family Physicians. 2006; 55: 1-3.

Last fall, as I visited each of our residencies and Family Medicine interest groups, I asked participants to complete a survey sharing their attitudes about what was most important to them in choosing treatment for their patients. They ranked each of the 10 items shown in table 1 from 1= least important to 5= most important. We had used these same surveys with our summer students including pre-med Trover Rural Scholars and UL medical students just before their M-1 year (Prematriculation Program) and just after the M-1 year (Preclinical Program). These programs are described in more detail in a recent publication (1) and on our web site (2). We also placed this survey as a tear-out in a recent journal issue, hoping some practicing family doctors would give us their opinions.

The 10 items can be grouped roughly into issues of basic science, clinical science, a business issue, spirituality, and patient ethnicity. Our expectation was that students would most value whatever they were studying at the time, with those further along in training placing more emphasis on health benefits and ethnicity. We didn't know what to expect on the issues of spirituality and the role of prayer, as this is less frequently discussed among physicians-in-training. The spiritual issues consistently ranked near the bottom of the priority rank among all participants. Interestingly, understanding the patient's ethnic background was ranked only slightly above these two spiritual issues.

Duke University's Harold Koenig, M.D. speaks regularly concerning religion, spirituality, and medicine (3). He summarizes the literature that makes the case that religion is relevant to health and that most U.S. patients, when facing important treatment decisions, want to discuss this issue with their doctors. In one study, 66% of patients indicated that their religious beliefs would influence their medical decisions. How many of us would choose not to ask about something so important to our patients? The literature says we don't.

I think often we doctors are so careful not to use our position of authority to proselytize that we risk ignoring an important part of our patients' lives. Dr. Koenig summarizes the elements of a spiritual history (see table 2)(4), as well as some techniques to avoid (see table 3). Nowhere is this more delicate than the question of when/if to pray with patients. In our summer sessions, this topic generated the liveliest discussions. Dr. Koenig suggests that shared prayer is most recommended when the patient and doctor share a similar religion, the patient requests it, and the situation warrants it. Our hospital chaplain shares some interesting stories about what happens just after he says the words "can we pray together?" Sometimes there's a prolonged silence, sometimes a clear prayer leader emerges, and sometimes everyone in the family begins praying out loud simultaneously. I guess that even among similar folks, prayer has no hard and fast rules.

It seems that just when I'm getting the most tired and cynical, a patient jolts me back to why I chose to do this in the first place. Seeing the simple strength of their faith in the face of overwhelming stress is their witness to me. Ministry goes both ways.

It has been an honor to be your President.

### *Table One*

Indicate your opinion concerning the importance of understanding the following items in choosing the best treatment for your patient.

1. Biochemical Abnormality
2. Anatomy
3. Role of spirituality in the patient's life
4. Laboratory abnormalities
5. Imaging (x-ray, ultrasound, etc.) abnormalities
6. Health benefits held by the patient
7. Mechanism of medications used
8. Role of prayer in the patient's life
9. Published expert guidelines
10. Ethnic background of the patient's family

## Table Two

Spiritual History

Introduction is necessary (why asking these questions):

1. Do religious/spiritual beliefs provide comfort or cause stress?
2. How might beliefs influence medical decisions?
3. Are there beliefs that might interfere/conflict with medical care?
4. Member of a religious/spiritual community & is it supportive?
5. Any other spiritual needs that someone should address?

## Table Three

What is Not Recommended

1. Prescribe religion to non-religious patients.
2. Force a spiritual history if patient not religious.
3. Coerce patients in any way to believe or practice.
4. Spiritually counsel patients.
5. Any activity that is not patient-centered.
6. Argue with patients over religious matters (even when it conflicts with medical care/treatment)

## References

1. Crump WJ, Fricker S, Barnett D. A Sense of Place: Rural training at a regional medical school campus. Journal of Rural Health. 2004;20(1):80-84.
2. www.troverfoundation.org/octc.
3. www.heritage.org/emails/hidden/koenig_presentation.ppt
4. Koenig HG. An 83-year-old woman with chronic illness and strong religious beliefs. JAMA. 2002;288(4):487-93.

**Crump WJ. The Future Of Family Medicine: A View From The Commonwealth's Blacktops. Journal of the Kentucky Academy of Family Physicians. 2006; 55: 3-4.**

During my year as KAFP president, I traveled across our state and visited all our residency training programs and student interest groups. As I drove back from each visit, I had a chance to reflect on my impressions. I shared some of these with our annual banquet attendees as my Presidential Address, and I'll do the same here in text. A recurring impression was that our discipline is at a crossroads. The sentiments of cynicism and idealism kept popping up as a dichotomy among old and young alike: Which shall we be? On several of my visits, I invited participants to provide some phrases to describe the successful physician. Among the most cynical, I heard things like "the nicest car in the doctor's lot," or the "trophy spouse."

For a lot of years, I have worked with bright young pre-med students just before they begin medical school, and I am continually impressed with their eager idealism. When I see the same students after the first year of medical school, something has changed, and cynicism is the rule. This reminds me of a quote from Dr. Rachel Remen's book (1):

"Medical training is like a disease. It would be years before I would recover from mine."

## CYNICISM

So let's think about cynicism for a bit. For a definition, let's turn to Wikipedia (2). A Cynic is someone who maintains that only self-interest motivates human behavior, and tends to dismiss most of accepted wisdom as irrelevant or obsolete nonsense. They view themselves as enlightened free-thinkers, with their critics seen as social pretenders who bury their heads in the sand.

But, too much cynicism may cause psychological distress when cynics see themselves as self-serving inhabitants of a meaningless, shallow world. One view is that excess cynicism lends to dissociation from reality because it leads to easy rejection of hard answers. To support their view, cynics point to media reports of misdeeds of politicians, corporations, and some organized religions. In fact, mass market journalism generally accepts only cynicism as the politically correct view (2).

Now a little about the history of cynicism (3): The Greek word Kynikos means "like a dog." The first cynics were students of the philosopher Antisthenes, who was a student of Socrates. Their goal was to expose foolishness. They hung out in the streets like a pack of dogs, watch the passing crowds, and ridiculed anyone who seemed pompous or pretentious.

Probably the most famous cynic was Diogenes who would introduce himself as follows. "I am Diogenes the dog. I nuzzle the kind, bark at the greedy, and bite scoundrels." His famous use of a lantern to search for an honest man was actually done during daylight hours to make his point. When Alexander the Great came upon Diogenes sitting in the market place and asked how he could help the old man, Diogenes is quoted as saying "You can step out of my sunlight." More modern cynics include Rabelais, Swift, Voltaire, and Mark Twain. Their common technique is biting sarcasm and mirthful ridicule.

## IDEALISM

So what about Idealism? Idealists pride themselves on being loving, kindhearted, and authentic. The table lists some common preferences of those who would call themselves idealists (4). A definition, again from Wikipedia: Idealism is a philosophy, or understanding of existence, that is the opposite of materialism (5). It's not really about being greedy or not- it's whether the world is a better understood as mental (idealism) or physical (materialism). In its purist form idealism says that the only things which can be directly known for certain are ideas. This is a very spiritual way of thinking, and is interwoven into most of the world's religions.

## CONCLUSION

So, what's all of this got to do with being a family doctor? Think back to when you made the decision to go to medical school- most of us were idealists, I think. So, what happened? This may be best explained by a quote from Rick Bayan, who manages the website The Cynic's Sanctuary (3):

"But the best cynics are still idealists under their scarred hides. We wanted the world to be a better place, and we can't shrug off the disappointment when it lets us down. Our cynicism gives us the painful power to behold life shorn of its sustaining illusions. Thus my own definition of a cynic: 'an idealist whose rose-colored glasses have been removed, snapped in two and stomped into the ground, immediately improving his vision.'

If we were activist, we'd do something constructive about our discontentment. But we're smart enough to know that we won't prevail, and probably a little too lazy to attempt any labor that's predestined to fail. So we retaliate with our special brand of wounded wit. If we can't defeat our oppressors, at least we can mock them in good fellowship. That's about as much justice as a cynic can expect."

Opponents of the cynical view say that cynicism is bad for the soul and leads to an unhappy life. When one begins to believe the view of the world provided by the media as mankind as a whole morally corrupt, it's hard to be enthusiastic about our future. This logically leads to burn-out, and we've all seen too much of that. What are we to do?

My mentor at Vanderbilt, Dr. Anderson Spickard, published a summary of the literature on burnout in JAMA (6). So which shall we be: cynic or idealist? On my travels I also heard phrases describing the successful physician in entirely non-materialistic terms. Phrases like those in Dr. Rick Miles' essay in this issue. Words like "blessed" and "energized" that were framed by the sheer wonder of the experience of caring for folks from birth to death.

Lastly, let me say that I can spend this time pondering the meaning of life because I know I have the leadership and advocacy of the AAFP "sweating the details" of practical, material gains for Family Medicine. Our future is bright, but only if each one of us agrees to spend our time in roles of leadership, getting up to our ears in the mire of payment mechanisms and politics. But I urge us to retreat to our idealism regularly. Only then can we be fully present with our patients who daily share their lives with us. Thank you.

## References

1. Remen RN. Kitchen table wisdom: Stories that heal. Riverhead Books. New York. 1996.
2. http://en.wikipedia.org/wiki/Cynicism
3. http://www.i-cynic.com/whatis.asp
4. http://www.ptypes.com/idealist.html
5. http://en.wikipedia.org/wiki/Idealism
6. Spickard A, Gabbe SG, Christensen JF. Mid-career burnout in generalist and specialist physicians. JAMA 2002;288:1447-50.

**Crump WJ. A Modest Proposal: Shorten Medical School and Produce More Family Doctors? Journal of the Kentucky Academy of Family Physicians, 2006; 56: 2-3.**

One of the roles of a journal editor is to create intellectual curiosity and stimulate reasonable controversy, so here goes. One of the things I do as a "Deanlet" of a medical school is to read the journal of the Association of American Medical Colleges (AAMC) <u>Academic Medicine</u>. The AAMC is considered the authoritative national voice of medical educators, and is generally perceived as fairly conservative. Clearly this organization is entrusted with the legacy of Louisville's Abraham Flexner to seek the highest quality for American medical education.

Recently the AAMC has begun to make strides into what we called in south Georgia "tall grass"- those issues likely to seem quiet from a distance but with lots going on underneath. Several months ago the lead editorial in their newsletter suggested that US medical educators should begin to learn more about offshore medical school training, since so many of our residents in training are their graduates. This is a bit of a departure from the traditional view that it might be best to ignore what are considered inferior institutions.

In the March 2006 Academic Medicine issue, the lead editorial broached another controversial topic, shortening medical school training to 3 years (1). This reconsideration of an old idea is based on the startling report that 60% of medical school matriculants come from families in the top 20% of income. There is accumulating evidence that many college students (including those that would fit the profile of students who choose Family Medicine and ultimately practice in underserved areas) give up on the idea of medical school for financial reasons.

In the same issue, an original report summarized the recent changes and 4 methods to address the issue (2). From 1990 to 2003, medical school tuition and fees increased 167%, and in 2003 the average debt for graduating students was $100,000. More recent anecdotal information is that the average now is closer to $120,000. Those of us close to medical students in training have seen another change during this time. Fewer medical students seem willing to delay "living like doctors," buying nice homes and nicer cars during medical school. While this lifestyle clearly doesn't represent those destined to be family doctors, it does add to the reported total indebtedness that may scare off college students from families of modest means.

The 4 methods reviewed by the article and the median net savings to the individual student shown in parentheses included: reducing tuition ($30,000), decreasing duration of medical school to 3 years ($200,000), increasing residency compensation ($80,000), and decreasing residency duration for medical subspecialists ($170,000). The actual median values will likely be lower for primary care physicians because the model factors in first-year practice income, but the comparisons are still relatively valid.

So, what if? The ABFM model from many years ago combined medical school and FM residency into a 6 year program at selected sites, including UK in Lexington and Marshall in West Virginia. The perception of outsiders was that this was a very successful program, generating a not-so-small amount of jealousy in residency directors competing with these sites that seemed to have an "inside track" to some of the best students.

This 3+3 pilot program was allowed only for FM and Internal Medicine, and was ended in 2004 by the ACGME by a narrow interpretation of the requirement that residents must have graduated from medical school. There were many who believed that this was accomplished by specialties and sites excluded from the pilot program. The AAFP felt so strongly that this option should continue that last year, the Commission on Education sent a letter to the ACGME outlining the specific wording in Section VIII of the ACGME program requirements that should allow for continued approval of these innovative programs. Some believe that the timing is right for this change now.

If we re-created that system and all the assumptions held, it could: 1) attract more college students of modest means into medical school and ultimately into Family Medicine residencies in our Commonwealth, 2) guarantee our residencies a regular flow of American graduates where each student is a "known quantity" and 3)create innovative opportunities for programs that train medical students in regional community sites to collaborate with residencies in their region to ensure a seamless transition.

For instance, current M-4 requirements for Neurology or Anesthesia could be interwoven into some M-3 and some PG-1 experiences, to be sure the objectives were met. Some PG-1s in this new system would require more educational support (similar to that many programs are reporting with current offshore grads), a need that could be met best by medical school educators. In fact, rather than "retrofitting" once a PG-1 is determined to have special needs, it would be logical to address this during the M-3 year of a student in the 6-year Pathway. This has to be better than the current situation where our best residencies are scrambling to meet the unpredictable needs of offshore grads during the high pressure PG-1 year.

So what are the potential negatives of this new system? Certainly it would place even more pressure on young folks to make lifelong decisions at younger ages. No later than beginning of the M-3 year, these students would have to be in this special track. What if they decide they want to change specialties to one not offering the 6-year option? Will they feel trapped by their financial commitments? What if family obligations limit their geographical choices for residency? One of my reasons for writing this editorial is to try to get feedback from M-1s and M-2s (and maybe even some pre-meds) who read our journal on how important these concerns are to them. We all have known students who at age 21 are ready to make such choices, as well as some who struggle at age 26.

I also want to hear from practicing docs and our academic leaders. Is this an innovative idea whose time is now or is this just crazy? Please write or Email me. I hope to get some responses that we can publish in future issues of our journal.

## *References*

1. Whitcomb ME. Who will study medicine in the future? Acad Med 2006;81:205.

2. Dorsey ER, Ninic D, Schwartz JS. An evaluation of four proposals to reduce the financial burden of medical education. Acad Med 2006;81:245-251.

## Crump WJ. What if Family Doctors were paid for tending the Medical Home? Journal of the Kentucky Academy of Family Physicians. 2007; 57: 3-5.

As I pondered the topic for my editorial for this issue, 2 articles in JAMA a week apart caught my eye. The first was a Commentary promoting changes in the systems we work in (1) and the other was a news summary of the recent publication of an international physician summary done by the Commonwealth Fund (2). The latter noted that physicians in the U.S. lag far behind other industrialized countries in the use of electronic health records (EHR) and arrangements for after-hours access by patients, excluding the Emergency Department (ED). Any time U.S. physicians are lumped together for ridicule, it both gets my interest and raises my ire (see Dr. Klein's letter to the editor in this issue). Usually, if I put the emotions aside, there's a kernel of truth in what the writer has to say.

Next some random comments to me from my mentors entered my head. I remember when I was in Steve Spann's department in Galveston, his comment in 1993: The enduring symbol of the physician is undoubtedly the stethoscope. In the next millennium, the primary care physician must be as facile with the computer, as managing information will be as important as hearing heart and lung sounds. And from Gayle Stephens, one of Family Medicine's founding fathers, in 1981: The mark of a family doctor is that we do not have the privilege of ignoring any complaint brought to us by our patients, whether it be medical, social, or administrative. And further, you become someone's personal physician when you can hear only their name and conjure up the fullness of that individual in your head.

Next I thought about my regular frustration when I try to force what I do with a patient into ICD-9 and CPT codes. The "bullets" in E and M coding include things like review of systems that every experienced clinician knows are nearly worthless, and parts of the physical exam that are so non-specific we learned long ago to ignore them (after carefully recording them so we can support a 99214). Decision-making is included in the template, but the writers mean interpreting lab and x-ray, mostly.

What family docs do that is priceless is help our patients manage their lives. When their concern is a teenager out of control or an impending job loss, we care. After a few years of practice in the real world, we realize that GERD and depression/anxiety are nice labels that don't begin to express the richness of human distress. There's an old quote that goes: "There's a reason that a general surgery residency lasts 5 years. It only takes a year to learn how to enter the abdomen safely, but it takes another 4 years to learn when not to." Similarly, the mark of a good personal physician is to know when not to consult for the chest pain, or when the best agent for the "soul pain" is not a narcotic or NSAID.

The JAMA commentary points out lessons learned from the fast food industry. The way to increase efficiency is not to cajole the staff to work harder and faster, but to change the system around them to make their job easier. We physicians are receiving plenty of advice on working harder and faster, when what is needed is fundamental change in the way we help our patients. A system that was designed to manage short duration acute illnesses simply can't work for the many chronic diseases we manage today.

The commentary recommended:

*1) Make it easier for patients to get access to care and obtain continuity.*

Studies have shown that patient and physician satisfaction, as well as the rate of preventive services provided, increase when continuity is the routine. Consider the last time that you made decisions about a patient you didn't know well-it's a qualitatively different task. The focus currently is on easier access to an appointment, and this is important. Perhaps, though, the patient's need could be addressed without an office visit. And maybe it could be met just as well by your nurse or another staff member who knows your routines.

Imagine if the revenue you received was not dependent on seeing the patient in the office. Although capitation is no longer in vogue, my practice in Texas in the 1990s discovered a different office system that is made possible by capitation. Being paid the same per member per month whether you saw them or not meant that keeping most patients out of the office and keeping the precious office slots full with those who needed in-person help managing their lives was a "win-win," and we did well financially. We invested our group's time in establishing protocols for the things we saw repeatedly and training our office staff on the protocols. Eventually we were large enough to pay a nurse to answer our calls at night, using the protocols to get the patient through until their personal physician could make the long-term decisions. Our patients rarely insisted on speaking with the doctor, once they knew that our staff was speaking for us and that they could get in to see us easily when it was really needed.

## 2) Find ways to increase the patient's participation in their care

Studies show that often the patient's agenda is not fully addressed in the typical office visit. Attention so far has focused on training the doctor to be better at discerning the patient's agenda (i.e., work harder and faster). Shifting some of the responsibility to the patient has been shown to be successful. In some settings "agenda cards" with the most common issues of each clinical condition are provided to patients, either on paper or electronically. In advance of the visit, patients sort through and prioritize what's important to them at that time, increasing the efficiency of the visit. The current attention being given to electronic personal health records may be a way to maximize this process. When a patient has an opportunity to review (and offer corrections to) her medical history, including family history, active illnesses, and medications, she can be empowered to be her own health advocate. The best of these systems allow only the doctor to make changes, facilitating the "negotiation" that should go on before a medical history is finalized.

## 3) Provide the skills necessary for patient self-care

The commentary points out that patient education in the traditional sense is not enough to get patients to make the lifestyle changes that are critical to their health. Tangible skills must be learned, practiced, and become part of everyday life. An often successful technique is individual patient-to-patient interaction or group activities where actual skills are taught. I remember that by far the best way for me to promote weight loss in my patients in one of my practice sites was to connect each with one of my patients who facilitated a weekly weight loss group in her home. Not only did they learn the particulars of "counting points," but they had a ready support group when the inevitable back-sliding begins. Another example was a practice that put some exercise machines in an unused area of the office, allowing staff and patients to use them at no charge in the evening, even paying for healthy snacks and providing bottled water on "team night."

## 4) Coordinate care among different clinical settings

We all have had situations where a consultant repeated a test or misunderstood our question because of poor communication, or the ED admitted a patient because they didn't have access to a previous EKG or chest radiograph. For now, having a standard referral/consultation form is helpful, and EHRs shared by multiple points of care solve many of these problems. The ultimate frustration of having a patient go to an academic referral center and then return to see us before we receive any information about their stay is less common now. The Neonatology group I use most frequently simply faxes me the computer-generated note on my patient each Friday that lists all the active problems and the status of each. It is very reassuring to the new mother's family that I can explain how things are going in laymen's terms. Our own multi-specialty group has multiple-point access to lab, imaging, and office and hospital notes now, and it has saved me hours of chasing lab or consultants and allows me to explain the results face-to-face during the patient's office visit.

When I reflect on these recommendations, I am struck with just how modern our student-led free clinic has become. We have a very simple EHR, and can access all the reports from our multi-specialty group's system from multiple points. When I attend the students there, it seems so easy: since payment is not an issue, we can just do the history, physical, and lab that are really needed, throwing coding templates out the window. We have just begun a project of assigning these patients to a student for continuity of care. Freed from the need for office visits just to allow billing, we can see these patients less frequently, managing their chronic diseases "virtually" by telephone. Our nurse communicates with the students and me by Email, allowing us to choose the most convenient time to answer and begin the next step of management. We will be able to communicate with some of these patients directly by Email, as they can get access from a public library or a friend's house. This would include reminders to come together for group skills sessions or individual foot exams, as well as when to go to the lab. The results of the self blood glucose monitors we provide for our diabetics can be downloaded electronically, allowing us to make those decisions without seeing the patient. All of these patients are working uninsured, so this not only saves them time but allows us to serve many more patients, less limited by our brief weekly clinic sessions.

So, imagine how your practice may look in the New Virtual Care World, where you are paid for helping to manage your patients' lives, regardless of how frequently you see them. With well-developed office systems allowing your staff to do much of what you do now, you could actually spend that extra time with that patient on the day he needs it. Most projections have actually shown that a physician in this model should be able to manage about 10-20% more lives without increasing staff or clinic hours. And in this model, covered lives equals revenue.

I invite comments on this version of the brave New Virtual Care World. Are you ready for this?

## References

1. Bergeson SC, Dean JD. A Systems Approach to Patient-Centered Care. JAMA 2006;296:2848-51.
2. Mitka M. Electronic Health Records, After-Hours Care Lag in US Primary Care Practices. JAMA 2006:296:2913-4.

**Crump WJ. Speak with one voice: Our Commonwealth needs more Family Doctors. Journal of the Kentucky Academy of Family Physicians. 2007; 58: 3-4.**

The leadership of your Academy attended a 4-hour workshop recently to understand the workforce needs of Kentucky. Within the mission of the KAFP, our focus was on improving the health of our population while promoting family medicine as the foundation for healthcare in the commonwealth. The national perspective was brought by Dr. Amy McGaha, with the AAFP Medical Education Department. The scope and work plan of the Kentucky Institute of Medicine to address this issue was presented by the Director, Dr. Emery Wilson, and his staff. The KMA, through funding made available by the Kentucky Rural Scholarship Foundation, Inc., has tasked the KIOM to report their findings by August, and this meeting was the initiation of a process to ensure that the voice of the KAFP is heard.

Referring to a recent report, an expert at a recent Association of American Medical Colleges (AAMC) workforce meeting made two points. First, there is currently a physician shortage, and second, it's here to stay. He suggested both that medical schools produce more doctors and that residencies create more positions. The AAFP recently sponsored a study done by the University of Utah School of Medicine that used current assumptions to project the numbers of family physicians needed in each state by 2020. By this method, Kentucky will need 555 new family doctors within the next 14 years. That's roughly 40 FM resident graduates per year, if they all stayed in Kentucky. Currently, about 64% of our resident grads stay here, and that percentage is much lower for physicians who are not native Kentuckians.

We currently provide 36-39 first-year positions in the match, so that means that we will need to: 1) add more resident slots, and 2) do a better job of filling these with Kentuckians. The larger problem is at the medical school level. In a good year, our 2 allopathic schools match 25 graduates into Family Medicine, with about half staying in Kentucky. So although ultimately more resident slots are needed, the more urgent problem is filling the slots we have with physicians likely to stay in Kentucky. There is also an important maldistribution of physicians in Kentucky, with 61%

of our counties (73 of the 120) considered underserved now. So we need to admit persons to medical school who are more likely to choose small town practice.

So where do we start? Dr. McGaha recommends a 3-pronged approach. First, recruit the right students into family medicine. Second, train them in residencies that prepare them for Kentucky practice, with more prepared for rural practice. And third, work to enhance the practice environment to retain these physicians in practice in Kentucky.

## RECRUITMENT

Many studies have shown that facilitating medical school entry for college students from small towns with an interest in service as a strong motivating factor will result in more family physicians in small towns in the native state. The issue in Kentucky is the very small applicant pool, with perhaps only 2 in-state applicants for each medical school position, with the vast majority of those being students from metropolitan areas. So, nothing of substance can change without getting more successful applicants from small towns. Despite education reform, small town high schools do not routinely prepare students for success in premedical curricula. Most studies have shown that although small town students start out behind those from metro areas in almost every standardized measure of academic performance, this difference disappears during medical school.

So how do we get these targeted students the boost they need to get into medical school and be successful by the time they take Step One (basic science) Board exams? Dr. McGaha summarized the Alabama Rural Medical Scholars program that provides a fifth undergraduate or post-baccalaureate year for selected students, and they have placed 50% of their graduates into rural practice. We have the 3-year, summers-only Trover Rural Scholar premedical program partially modeled after the Alabama program that has also been successful. Such programs will need to be replicated across our state for the recruitment issue to be addressed.

Another important issue is medical student indebtedness. As I discussed in a previous editorial, there is mounting evidence that the very students who would likely end up in Family Medicine are not choosing medical school because of the potential debt. To these students who have grown up largely in families of very modest means, incurring a debt of well over $100,000 is daunting. To address this issue, a much larger statewide program of loan repayment for practicing in an underserved area will be required.

## TRAINING

Once the right students succeed in the basic science years of medical school, they must enter a clinical environment that fosters their natural tendencies. This means longer FM clerkships, and as many rural experiences for as long as possible. A regional rural campus is the ultimate of this strategy, with the entire last 2 years spent in a supportive environment. The ULSOM Trover Campus has been active now for 9 years, based in Madisonville, a town of 20,000. To date about 50% of the grads have chosen family medicine, and 78% of rural students who have finished their residencies, regardless of specialty choice, have chosen small town practice. For a workforce plan to succeed, this model must be replicated across the state.

Once medical students graduate with their interest in FM intact, they must have residencies that build their confidence to practice where they're needed. Although less strong as a predictor than growing up in a small town, residency training in rural areas is associated with ultimate practice in an underserved location. But we will also need replacement of retiring family docs in metro areas, so all our residencies need to be strong and well-funded.

## RETENTION

Once we "get 'em there", we've got to "keep 'em there." Much of the daily activities of your AAFP and KAFP is to do just this. Successes are few and far between, but the last few months have brought cause for optimism. Nationally, the relative value of our most common office visits has been increased by 9-13%. Kentucky Medicaid has had the first increase in reimbursement for the common codes in almost 15 years, and the percentage increase is dramatic. The recent interest from IBM and other major employers in an efficient health system managed by generalists may just usher in the next golden era for Family Medicine.

## THE BOTTOM LINE

The KAFP Task Force will be meeting and working throughout the summer, and will bring recommendations back to the KAFP Board of Directors. Some of these recommendations, if endorsed, include regular action steps with the legislature to effect change. KAFP leadership will be in communication with members. It will be incumbent on us, with our personal contacts, to make the changes needed.

So, the next legislative session is likely to be busy with issues of physician workforce. We must speak with one voice. Unlike some disciplines that practice professional contraception, family docs have never been afraid of adding another of this special breed in their community – as long as we have enough to keep us busy. Certainly, all of our rural areas can accommodate more family docs. So, if a legislator (or anyone else) asks you: "So, do we need more doctors like you in Kentucky?" we hope you can respond with a resounding "Yes, especially in our rural areas." Comments appreciated.

**Crump WJ. How Do Doctors Think (And Feel)? Journal of the Kentucky Academy of Family Physicians. 2007; 59: 1-3.**

One of the special privileges of a journal editor is to write periodically about whatever is on his mind, hoping that readers will connect with the ideas. This is a fun time of year for me. I am interviewing bright young people who think they want to go to medical school and making the difficult decisions that go with that process. We recently completed our summer programs for college students and preclinical medical students where our focus is on learning to "think like a clinician." I have begun the year-long process that is "Dean's Hour" with our ten new third-year medical students who are with us in Madisonville for the last 2 years of med school. Much of that time is also spent getting these students to learn the iterative process of decision-making that is required for success in clinical medicine. So, I think a lot about how doctors think.

A recent AMA publication highlighted Dr. Jerome Groopman's book on this topic (1). Although I dove into this book with my usual energy, it was soon dissipated. He did a nice job outlining the kind of errors in thinking that can occur in clinical care, like the "closing too soon" that can occur when something about the patient causes us to rule in or out important diagnoses before we have enough information. But I have to admit that two things he did early in the book made me put it down prematurely. First, when listing the specialties and the thought patterns of each, he seems to have forgotten ours. I hope that this is just a reflection of the narrowness of his training. Second, he excludes behavioral/psychiatric illness from consideration. Excuse me, Dr. Groopman, but if you exclude these issues, the rest is really easy in comparison.

The other thing that concerns me about the sensationalism of his book is best summarized by an old aphorism. It is said that when an experienced clinician hears hoof beats, she thinks first of horses, and then zebras. This highlights the differences between probabilistic thinking (what's it most likely to be) and possibilistic thinking (everything it could possibly be).

We've all worked with inexperienced clinicians who do an MRI on the first 30 patients they see with tension headaches before they learn what that clomping sound on the turf represents. Much of FM residency training is unlearning the possibilistic thinking that is ingrained during most (sub-specialty driven) medical school education. Not only must we be good stewards of the health care dollars that COULD be spent looking for striped horses, but many tests themselves are uncomfortable and invasive. We must be our patient's advocate.

For instance, the 24 year-old with anxiety and abdominal pain COULD have a colonoscopy, but a 54 year-old with a family history of colon cancer in young relatives SHOULD have one. A personal reflection on this issue comes from my current study in preparation for my every- ten-year recertification exam in Geriatrics. I am using the most highly recommended set of texts that, unfortunately, were written by possibilistic thinkers. A common clinical scenario is spun, and the "right" answer is a very rare condition. These kinds of texts are especially dangerous for beginners, because they don't know any better. At least I know that if I've never seen a condition after 13 years in major medical centers and 25 years of community practice (sometimes overlapping), that's probably not the real correct answer in the scenario. So, my plan is to choose mostly zebra answers on the test and then go back to working with horses in my daily practice – I just hope the exam answers are written by possibilists this time.

I heard a story in medical school at Vandy that a professor of Infectious Diseases was truly impressed with a "local MD" who sent a patient in to a medical center with a correct diagnosis of a liver echinococcal cyst. This was long before the days of CT scans. The intern who had admitted the patient was unimpressed, as he had seen some of the patients who this same doctor sent in almost monthly with the same incorrect diagnosis. It seems that in the mind of this doc, everyone in his town with right upper quadrant pain was (incorrectly) assumed to have been eating worm eggs, and after years of unnecessary referrals, he finally got one right. This is the epitome of possibilistic thinking.

Perhaps the most important part of the aphorism, though, is "…and THEN zebras." The mark of a good clinician is detecting that patient who, among all the common illnesses we see every day, just doesn't fit the usual profile. There was the young woman I saw who had mild shoulder pain when she became supine and was a little dizzy when standing who later was found to have 3 units of blood in her peritoneal space from a ruptured ectopic pregnancy. She reported a "normal" menstrual period 3 weeks before (a decidual reaction), no history of STDs (the bloody fimbria was pristine at the time of surgery), and no recent intercourse (as it turned out, by her definition of recent). For some reason that is difficult to put into words, I did not let her entirely unimpressive abdominal and pelvic exam sway me into sending her home with a potentially life-threatening condition.

So the good clinician dwells in probabilistic thinking and is able to switch to possibilistic just in time. Groopman's book highlights case after case where probabilistic thinking caused serious errors, and I think this is misleading to the lay reader. Folks don't buy books that detail the many correct diagnoses made every day using the probabilistic method. And actually, I worry less about the way docs think than I do about how they feel about patient care. There is much emphasis on "professionalism" in medical schools these days, and it is energy well-spent. Some readers may remember my penchant for quoting from Dr. Rachel Remen's "Kitchen Table Wisdom" book that was the basis for the "Doctoring 101" course that we teach during our summer programs (2). This summer, at the suggestion of a student, we substituted "Soul of a Doctor" that is a group of essays written by Harvard clinical medical students (3). A quote from one of these medical students may help frame this important issue:

"Physicians are taught to be doers. Directing patient interviews, examining the body, performing procedures, and prescribing medications constitute the bulk of the job description in today's world of medicine. Listening, perhaps seen as a more passive activity, seems undervalued and tends to get lost in the shuffle. No box exists to check "Listened" on the reimbursement form (not that I would advocate financial valuation of listening). Undoubtedly the "doer" elements form a vital part of both healing and meeting the expectations of patients. But I sense that medicine could mean and be much more for patients if time spent listening to the patient tell his or her story were prized. Might that mean longer patient visits? Possibly.

Others will write this off as the ravings of a naive, optimistic medical student; the advocates of efficient health care will be quick to argue that longer patient visits are not "cost effective." While that may be, we cannot forget medicine's fundamental premise that patients matter most. Complaints about the frantic pace and lack of human compassion in medicine commonly fill the general public's conversation about health care. The patients who sue their doctors for medical mistakes are the same ones who feel ignored and disregarded by their physicians.

In fact I would argue that in the long run, a reinvigorated emphasis on listening to the patient would be cost effective. I suspect that greater emphasis on hearing the patient's perspective could lead to improved diagnosis, patient understanding of their illness, and patient compliance with medications and preventive practices. All of which would likely lead to a patient population with improved health and fewer patient visits, thus alleviating overcrowded clinics and reducing health care costs."

Another book I can recommend that addresses professionalism from a spiritual perspective is written by a Franciscan Friar who is a physician (4). A brief quote summarizes his view:

"The human body is the place where human life and human love happen. The crafts of medicine, nursing, dentistry, and all the other healing arts require at least two human bodies-that of the healer and that of the one who is healed. It is in human bodies that the spirit of God transforms the air we merely breathe into the grace of God that touches every cell in our mortal bodies, forms any words of Good News we will ever proclaim, and moves us to works of charity and worship."

This perspective is also eloquently summarized in the Residency Graduation Prayer that is republished as a postscript in this book (see below). It reminds us that however we think, we must feel the call to service that is medical practice. Your comments are appreciated.

### *References*

1. Groopman J. How Doctors Think. Houghton Mifflin, Boston. 2007
2. Remen RN. Kitchen Table Wisdom. Riverhead Books, New York. 1994.
3. Pories S, Jain SH, Harper G. The Soul of a Doctor: Harvard medical students face life and death. Algonquin Books, Chapel Hill, NC. 2006.
4. Sulmasy DP. A Balm for Gilead. Georgetown University Press, Washington DC. 2006

# *A RESIDENCY GRADUATION PRAYER*
(St. Vincent's Hospital-Manhattan)

All powerful, all holy, all loving

Good and gracious God,

We thank you and we praise you for the privilege of caring for the sick;

For the mysterious beauty of the human body which you have created;

For the gifts of the earth by which we heal;

For the power of your presence in our professional lives.

We ask your grace that we may never consider our intelligence to be sufficient without fervor;

Knowledge without awe;

Counseling without respect;

Examination without reverence;

Diagnosis without meaning;

Prognosis without hope;

Therapy without compassion.

We pray that we may always be grateful to those who have taught us this art.

We pray together for the humility to remain students forever.

We pray today that you will bless our residents as they graduate,

That they may carry within themselves a little bit of this place of healing and learning wherever their careers may take them,

And that, in the spirit of St. Vincent de Paul, they may always hold a special place in their hearts for the sick and the poor of our world.

Amen.

## Crump WJ. Just Exactly What Does A Family Doctor do? Journal of the Kentucky Academy of Family Physicians. 2009; 63: 8-11.

As a new year begins, it is tradition to reflect on who we are, what we do, and what the new year might hold. As a dean of a regional medical school, I am asked some interesting questions. Just before the holiday break, as an M-3 medical student was headed out the door after final exams, he asked, expecting a quick answer: "So what is the difference between FM and IM/Peds?" In that same week, a pre-med student asked: "So what exactly do family doctors do?"

Our specialty has struggled with the answers to these questions for the entire 40 years of our modern re-incarnation. Dr. Kurfees in his editorial in this journal issue gives the view of one who has lived the answer. But how does one give a short answer? After all, OB/GYN is clearly the treatment of women only, Pediatrics is only children, and Internal Medicine is only adults. Urology is anatomically defined, as is gastroenterology and cardiology. My answer is clear, but not short. It's kind of like answering the old question: "So how do you recognize your mother in a crowd?" When you see her, you just know. When you see good family doctoring, you just know.

Family doctoring has less to do with specialty training than with attitude. Although I strongly believe that Family Medicine residency training is the most efficient way to discover the essentials of good doctoring, it is not necessary, nor sufficient. I have known and now practice among internists, pediatricians, and even an occasional surgeon or subspecialist who "get it." Also in almost 30 years of training Family Medicine residents, I realize that we are lucky if half of them leave our programs with "it," and even luckier if most of the other half learn it in practice in time to be good family doctors. So what is "it"?

One of the interesting things I get to do in my dean job is to read books about doctoring, choosing portions to share with the students in our pipeline programs, from high school through medical school. Two are pertinent to the "it" question. Although written primarily to a lay audience, Melissa Ramsdell's series of short essays from doctors of different specialties describing their first year of practice is truly insightful. (1)

From a family physician:

"It is easy to deal with objective disease entities and not deal with the human lives made complicated by disease. To do the latter requires that you get personal with your patients. Any personal relationship requires revealing something of yourself and stepping outside your clinical demeanor, something we are taught not to do in medical school. But it was unavoidable after spending time here with the people of eastern Kentucky. They have a way of disarming you with their unabashed realism, gentleness, and patience.... I rarely suffer from burnout anymore. Here, I learned that caring about people is the best medicine for my patients and for me."

From a general internist:

"By continually seeing people as their personal physician you can have an impact on their overall health. When you get to know them, it helps you influence them more.... It takes a special type of person to be patient with people and do preventive medicine. If you can get them to quit smoking, you've done something more important than doing a coronary bypass twenty years later, and certainly more cost-effective... Being able to sit down with them and listen to their problems is a privilege."

There are other interesting individual stories from the first year of practice in this book, but I was struck with something else. The hematologist/oncologist talked about helping a patient die, and the plastic surgeon described discovering something important beyond noses and breasts. Many of the "ologists" and other subspecialists worried aloud about being sued, and there was a clearly defined distance between them and their patients. And many, stated outright or between the lines, mused as to whether what they did made a real difference, or was just a good job in a weak economy. Herein lies some of what makes us different.

Good doctoring happens in that magical moment when the distance between the healer and the healed is suddenly bridged. There is much good talk these days of the value of the patient-centered medical home

(PCMH). I see this as an accounting method for good doctoring. If we do good things, our society should value our efforts, and we should be paid accordingly. As I tell my students, the day I am paid as much for working with a family in crisis as I am for delivering a baby, I will know that values have been properly realigned. As critically important as the new model is, PCMH is just details. It's like describing your mother's nose, and then her eyes, and then the way she holds her head cocked a bit when she first sees you. It's not the same as the process of recognition when you see her among all those other people. It is relationship-centered medical care that makes us different. Described in detail in 1994 (2), this concept is at the heart of good doctoring from my perspective.

Another book I'd recommend, but a much tougher read, is Jack Medalie et al's Life-changing stories from primary care (3). In the introduction to the section on Family and Community, Howard Brody fleshes out this concept of relationship-centered care. He points out that essentially every doctor-patient encounter is a cross-cultural event. Medical school is an acculturation to a different world view:

"Among the critical features of the exceedingly complex medical culture is a need to see the world as a composite of problems with solutions, where the "right" solution is often independent of which person has the problem. ...Hippocrates laid the groundwork for Western medicine by claiming that no disease was supernatural – that all diseases could be understood by the study of natural biological phenomena– he also laid the foundation for a medical practice in which the physician no longer feels the need to speak to the patient." This is the essence of what is not relationship-centered medicine. To be human is to be shaped inevitably by one's culture, but to be shaped in a way which is simultaneously and constantly influenced by our family background and by our own individual personality. No two people are members of a culture in quite the same way; simply knowing a list of cultural beliefs and practices is insufficient to understand how any individual within that culture will behave or what he or she will value."

Think about the last time you were able to understand your patient's issues quickly because you know his family of origin. You suppose that's why it's called Family Medicine? Brody goes on to summarize the 3 essential elements common to all healing practices in all cultures:

1. Provide a meaningful explanation for the illness
2. Express care and concern
3. Manage the possibility of mastery and control over the illness or its symptoms

Good doctoring means accomplishing those three tasks and this is impossible without solid, trusting relationships. "Perhaps…we could finally come to manage the education of future professionals properly if we could somehow put these nested relationships at the center of the experience of becoming a healer, and emphasize that all else-scientific knowledge, clinical skills, and so on – is critical precisely to the extent that it serves and extends those relationships." Philip Yancy, in his delightful treatise on the Christian concept of grace (another book I strongly recommend), reviews the sociologic concept of the looking-glass self (4). This view holds that you become what the most influential people in your life think you are. Could it be that our relationships with our patients actually define who we are as doctors?

So, far from being anti-scientific, this concept of good modern doctoring requires both good science and good listening.

"The centrality of relationship as a way of both knowing and healing in primary care brings us back again to the importance of local knowledge. One forms relationships not with abstractions, but with specific people, families, and communities. … even caring physicians dedicated to these relationships may fail, but physicians neglectful or dismissive of these relationships will almost certainly fail (3)." Is it any wonder that our current medical system in America fails so many of us?

The importance of local knowledge is almost second-nature to most Kentuckians. The geographer Cutchin, studying rural Kentucky physicians, reported that remaining in practice for longer periods was associated with finding meaning in the overarching concept of the sense of place (5). When seeking meaning, in addition to one's personal faith, it is the land, the families, and the community that provides the answers.

Whether rural or urban, primary care or subspecialist, it is understanding and appreciating the relationships of daily practice that define the good doctor. In my experience, a key difference between burned-out physicians and those who keep their enthusiasm for practice is this difference in attitude. The former are just "passing through" the community in which they live. The latter have deep roots, and understand that sense of place.

So how do we help students recognize our specialty in a crowd? Invite them to spend awhile with you. They'll get it. Comments appreciated.

## *References*

1. Ramsdell Melissa. My first year as a doctor. Penguin Books. New York, NY. 1996.

2. Tresolini CP, and the Pew-Fetzer Task Force on Advancing Psychosocial Health Education (P-FTF). Health professions education and relationship-centered care. San Francisco. Pew Health Professions Commission. 1994

3. Borkan J, Reis S, Steinmetz D, and Medalie JH. Patients and Doctors. Life changing stories from primary care. The University of Wisconsin Press. Madison, WI. 1999.

4. Yancey Philip. What's so amazing about grace? Zondervan Publishing House. Grand Rapids, MI. 1997.

5. Cutchin MP. Physician retention in rural communities: the perspective of experiential place integration. Health Place. 1997;3:25-41.

*The summer of 2009 marked an inflection point for Dr. Crump. His youngest daughter had begun medical school in his home institution the year prior. He had shared closely in her immersion in an evangelical Christian youth group in college, and much of his outside reading was chosen based on what she was reading. When she was in her first year of medical school at the urban campus, he for the first time heard through her ears and saw through her eyes the concerns of preclinical medical students. This was reflected in the essays of this time. During 2009, a new dean in Louisville began a medical history course for the preclinical students. Always seriously interested in history, Dr. Crump committed to auditing the course, reading the assignments and listening to the recorded lectures. This changed his perspective on the practice of medicine and highlighted the key errors of the dogma of each time, from Hippocrates to the present. While still focused on the policy issues of the day, this historical perspective became interwoven among the essays that followed.*

## Crump, WJ. Mechanics, War, and Doctors. Journal of the Kentucky Academy of Family Physicians. 2009; 65: 5

As I reflect on the breadth of the articles in this month's journal issue, I am struck with something special about our discipline. As this idea forms in my head, I'm thinking about a radio segment I heard this AM that likened doctoring to the role a mechanic plays in our culture. The "car guy" is basically a businessman, and has information and understanding of our car's workings that the "lay" person doesn't have. So when he suggests that we need a $350 repair to keep us moving and safe, we tend to accept his recommendation. And then when the equivalent of the car MRI is completed, and something more significant is found, we swallow hard and come up with the additional $850 that's now required.

Even the radio commentators noted some differences between this analogy and modern American medicine. First, if the repairs cost more than we think the car is worth, we'd just scrap it. Despite talk show drivel that says otherwise, we're just not a country of euthanizers. The second difference is that the $1200 repair bill would likely just cost us about $150 to $250 in co-pay if we are privately insured, and zero if we're covered by automobile Medicaid. A trusted, knowledgeable person is recommending something that may save my car's life, and it seems like quite a bargain, so why not proceed?

This analogy generates something akin to nausea in me. How did we get here? The concept of health insurance began as accident and disability insurance around the time of the Civil War, and transitioned to sickness insurance around the time of the First World War (1). Employer-based health insurance that is tax exempt arose as a way for companies to attract scarce workers during World War 2, at a time when wages were frozen by law. Then came Medicare and Medicaid around the time of the Vietnam War. What is it about war time that is associated with health payment changes? Now we are fighting on two fronts in Iraq and Afghanistan, and we've decided we can't afford the health payment system we have. Both the left and the right of the political spectrum have staked out their territory. Will it end like the days of the Clinton plan of 15 years ago? Then there's the whole "businessman" thing. When did medicine transition from ministering to the needy to "providers" apportioning "services" to "consumers?" Historians argue, but I believe that something was lost when the "third parties" entered the exam room.

Back to what strikes me in this journal issue. Dr. French doesn't mention the business model in his carefully crafted letter to the editor. This despite the fact that data from Barbara Starfield summarized by the AAFP Graham Center makes the clear case that family physicians provide the best care with the lowest overall cost (2). And Dr. Calico's thoughtful summary of the new center in Danville talks about engaging the physician with the community and improving population health – neither of which have a CPT code nor payment associated with them. Drs. Wrightson and Stone describe fearlessly venturing into the mouths of toddlers to prevent caries, a scourge of our rural areas. Dr. Bennett's complete analysis of changes in Medicare payment for rural care highlights just how important these changes can be for family physicians.

So what strikes me is that family physicians simply do what needs to be done, where it needs to happen, without regard for specialty lines or whether it leads to personal gain. And our gaze goes beyond the walls of our offices and hospitals, to where our patients live. The modern John Snows point out the pump that spreads cholera (3) and the modern Maimonides consider that man can only seek God in His fullness when his basic health needs are met (4). The modern Semmelweis notes when the traditions of medical training may be harming more than they help (5).

So find some time, sit back, and enjoy this journal issue- you deserve it.

## *References*

1. Lumerer KM. Time to heal: American medical education from the turn of the century to the era of managed care. 1999. Oxford University Press. New York.

2. http://www.graham-center.org

3. Taylor RB. White coat tales: Medicine's Heroes, Heritage, and Misadventures. 2008. Springer Science + Media, LLC. New York.

4. Nuland SB. Maimonides. 2005. Schoken Books (Random House). New York.

5. Nuland SB. 2003. The doctors' plague: Germs, childbed fever, and the strange story of Ignac Semmelweis. WW Norton and Company. New York.

## Crump WJ. Returning to our roots: What skills are most needed to tend the medical home? Journal of the Kentucky Academy of Family Physicians. Fall 2010; 69: 6-8

I'm in a philosophical mood these days, so bear with me. Maybe it's that my daughter and several of her middle-school friends are now third-year medical students at our Campus and I'm getting a close-up view of the making of doctors. Or just that I'm tired of hearing us called providers and cost/revenue centers. This class of M-3s knows me well enough that I get an unusually unfiltered look into what they think is important in doctoring. Even though they're busy learning the best timing for an operation in gallstone pancreatitis and the controversy about drug-eluting stents for coronary disease, something in our last JKAFP issue stopped them in their tracks. The piece "Reach Out and Touch" from Dr. Eddie Prunty's article came at the right time for me, and at least for several of these students. I searched and also couldn't find who to attribute it to, so I'll just reference him (1) and repeat a bit of it here:

## REACH OUT AND TOUCH

Reach out your hand and touch me – if you dare. I am sick, afraid, insecure, fearful, apprehensive, lonely and misunderstood. I have no particular age, color, creed, or sex, but I share with others one particular emotion – fear of the unknown. I am a patient....

It's easy to love the lovely, but how about me – the dirty, smelly, unlovely bit of humanity that you see. My hair has never been styled in a beauty salon. I know so little of the niceties you enjoy, and I stand in awe of you in your immaculate white – so cool, sweet-smelling and secure. My world is different from yours. What do you know of near starvation and trying to rear six children on a pitiful amount of money, of no heat in the winter and outside toilets? "Anyone can stay clean," you say. Maybe in your world, but everything is more difficult in mine. It's easy for you to turn away. Don't reduce me still further. Touch my hand or my arm. Explain what's about to happen to me. Don't let me see the distaste in your eyes. Let me see instead your humility.

On and on we come – as unhappy children, misunderstood teenagers, elated new parents and tired old folks. We are all different, but our needs are exactly the same. Can you think of me as a person and not just a patient? Are you willing to smile when your feet hurt, to linger when you need to hurry, to always remain calm and unruffled? To keep offering the cup of kindness time and time again, even when it's not returned to you? Do you really care what happens to me, and is there enough of you to handle all the details of your job and still have time to show genuine concern for me? Do you love enough to reach out and touch me? I wonder.

How could any doctor, or really anyone, fail to be moved by these words? It's confusing being a doctor these days. When I'm seeing patients in our free clinic, I rediscover just how much fun it is to see patients. I don't have to worry about how many "bullets" I need to record to be able to code for a 99214. And I don't have to worry about how in the world I'm going to get this story of human misery collapsed down to fit an EMR template that requires categorization of the human experience. I don't have to worry about which drug formulary I must use for this patient- Wal Mart has most of what I really need. All I really have to do is connect with the patient and family in the room with me-really hear, really understand their concerns. Skip the Review of Systems, since I've never learned anything important from this futile exercise. Do a minimum of physical exam, because almost all I usually need to make a diagnosis is a good history. Do a minimum of lab, and almost no imaging, because it's unnecessary. There's no need for defensive medicine here. And our patients are truly appreciative.

The confusion begins when I leave this free clinic environment and re-enter the real world of modern primary care. There are just so many distractions to connecting – really connecting- with my patients and their families. In the past I've told students that if they're willing to make about half of the typical doctor's income and see about half the number of patients per day, they can practice this idyllic medicine. The distractions and digital noise all around us put even this model in jeopardy. As I contemplate what's next for primary care, I'm reminded of the words of Gayle Stephens, one of the "Founding Fathers" of Family Medicine. I was lucky enough to have him as an early mentor when I was a resident at UAB in the early 80s. These words from 30 years ago still ring true (2):

## A DECALOGUE FOR FAMILY PRACTICE RESIDENTS ENTERING PRACTICE

DON'T give up the reform ethos. Keep on the side of responsible change in education, practice, and social justice.

DON'T lose faith in the power of relationships and the therapeutic use of self. (Or, don't hire anybody to save you from spending time with patients.)

DON'T turn your practice into a mere business. It may not be less, and it should be a great deal more.

LEARN to distinguish between uncertainty and ignorance; only the latter is remediable and potentially culpable.

FIND some way to practice charity; i.e., willingly give a part of your services consistently to those who cannot pay.

TRY to see that the groups in which you hold membership are at least as moral as you are.

HUMANIZE and personalize the microsystems in which you work.

ACT at all times as if the patient is fully autonomous; the weaker the patient is, the more vulnerable you are to violating his/her personhood.

REFLECT on your professional experiences. Within the bounds of protecting patients' privacy, think, talk, and write about your clinical stories.

WORRY less about patients becoming overly dependent on you than about your becoming undependable.

G. Gayle Stephens

(Originally presented as part of an address to the Department of Family Practice, Medical University of South Carolina, June 1979.)(2)

I'm naturally an optimist. What is next for doctoring? It is my fondest wish that the Patient-Centered Medical Home allows us to practice the kind of medicine I describe above (3). Imagine if you were paid for keeping your patients healthy and could share their care when they need it with your office staff. The diabetic could get advice on medication changes from your nurse without having to see you, and the practice would still be paid. A group of your obese patients could visit in your office with one of your patients who has been successful losing weight while you were spending time with your family. A smoking cessation class also run by one of your patients could be going on while you are at your daughter's soccer game. Maybe even a 12-step meeting can occur in your office while you're at a birthday party. And your practice would be rewarded for it all.

But wait, are we breaking Dr. Stephens' 2nd rule? I think not. Imagine if, in addition to advising all your office staff and group leaders each day, all you had to do was see the 10-12 patients who really need YOU (not some nameless, faceless provider) that day. When their illnesses have come to the level of suffering and only someone with your training, your skills, and your deep understanding of them as a human being can help, you're there for them. You are freed from the repetitive management questions for routine chronic disease issues, and most importantly, freed from the documentation monster. You are paid the same regardless of how well or badly your note corresponds to some arbitrary coding template. Your notes are for you and other physicians again.

I hope that this new model allows us to Reach out and Touch in the way that we do best. When future medical students first dream about doctoring, this is what they hope to get up every morning to do, and I know this because of the very many personal statements I've read on med school applications. But something happens along the way, and many become technicians just tinkering with the human body and losing touch with the soul. Is this what my daughter and her classmates are out there learning as I write this? I sincerely hope not.

The PCMH may not bring my idyllic vision into reality, but it's certainly worth a try. Your comments are appreciated, and I'll close with a quote from Daniel Sulmasy, a general internist and Franciscan friar, from one of my favorite books (4):

"The human body is the place where human life and human love happen. The crafts of medicine, nursing, dentistry, and all the other healing arts require at least two human bodies-that of the healer and that of the one who is healed. It is in human bodies that the spirit of God transforms the air we merely breathe into the grace of God that touches every cell in our mortal bodies, forms any words of Good News we will ever proclaim, and moves us to works of charity and worship."

Let's go heal.

## *References*

1. Prunty ME. Message from the president. JKAFP. 2010;68:8

2. Stephens GG. The Intellectual Basis of Family Practice. Tucson, AZ. Winter Publishing. 1982, p 237.

3. http://fmignet.aafp.org/online/fmig/index/family-medicine/pcmh.html

4. Sulmasy DP. A Balm for Gilead. Washington, D.C. Georgetown University Press. 2006.

*The editorial beginning a new decade gave Dr. Crump an opportunity to reflect more deeply and predict the future. Some aspects of this editorial in the statewide journal read by all specialties are truly prescient. Telecommuting would be fully embraced in 2021 as he predicted, not knowing that it would require a worldwide pandemic to accelerate this change. The revolutionary changes to office practice he predicted may yet happen, if the incredible inertia involved with payment reform can be overcome. Other aspects of his predictions were more fanciful, but are slowly finding their way into modern medical practice.*

**Crump WJ. A Glimpse of Medical Practice in 2021. Journal of the Kentucky Medical Association. January 2011; 109: 12-14.**

As I considered the appropriate content for my first editorial since joining the JKMA Editorial Board, my good fortune of being the first in the new decade occurred to me. So I will take this opportunity to share some predictions of what medical practice might look like in the year 2021, 10 years hence. At this point my daughter and her classmates will be settling into their first few years of practice, and I will be contemplating what retirement might look like. Some of my ideas might seem a little like the Jetsons, but hopefully are closer to reality than fantasy.

First, let's take a look at our world at the beginning of the next decade. And I say world because by now the digital divide between some formerly rich and poor countries has largely disappeared. China, India, and several South American countries are ascendant, and most citizens have easy access to the second version of the Internet, making communication nearly transparent. The issue of wireless charging of batteries has been solved, freeing all from cords and making digital devices as small and light as desired. LCD technology has progressed to allow for malleable flat screens. Now, we can access information and entertainment from a device worn on the wrist, looking like something between a wristwatch and the forearm band worn by quarterbacks that holds the key plays for his team. A ready and sustainable market is guaranteed for these devices by marketing their fashion value first to pre-teens, and then to everyone else. Logically, one must have a version for every occasion. Beepers are now things of the distant past.

Many of the vehicles now in the doctors' parking lot are powered by fuel cells or are stylish, powerful versions of that older technology, the gas/electric hybrid. Most are largely auto-piloted, directed by choosing one's locations on the vehicle's GPS system. This allows commuters to be fully engaged with their digital devices, with the display projected onto the windshield in the line of driving vision. The driver's only interaction with the vehicle is to brake when necessary to override the auto-pilot, much like a cruise control from the old days.

Voice recognition software has blossomed, freeing everyone from the keyboard. Commands to the digital device as well as voice to text has become routine. Most communication is off-line, leaving text messages for the receiver to consider at her leisure, assimilate into other digital contexts, and return the message. The remarkable comparison of this process with the antiquated voice mail technology is lost on my daughter's children as they snap up each new innovation. There is a key difference though, in that existing digital information can easily be inserted into these voice-to-text interactions, adding significant value to each.

Lastly, I predict that telecommuting will become more routine. Virtual meetings have become so lifelike that the in-person meeting sharing the same pastries and coffee is only a monthly event. This work routine removes some of the need for all office workers to be clustered in cities, allowing for the terms suburb and rural to merge. This routine also allows each of the monthly meetings to become mini-retreats. If workers are going to drive an hour each way, a several hour truly interactive process must replace the meeting where routine communications occur.

So where is medical practice in 2021? Most health care payment reforms have settled out, and a few real changes in daily practice have become established. My vision of this is based on the changes suggested by the Institute of Medicine report that by this time have had nearly 20 years to work their way into practice, as medical schools slowly began to prepare their graduates for the new world (1). The report suggests five competencies for medical professionals:

1. Provide patient-centered care
2. Work in interdisciplinary teams
3. Employ evidence-based practice
4. Apply quality improvement
5. Utilize informatics

In 2021, primary care practices are drastically different. As the manager of the medical home, primary care physicians have fewer exam rooms and more group spaces. Extended hours and same-day scheduling are facilitated by a truly interdisciplinary work group. Freed from the "piece work" payment method that rewards only a face-to-face encounter with the physician, primary care docs are paid a fixed amount to care for their population of patients, regardless of how this care is provided. Routine adjustments of medications and lab monitoring are managed largely using telephone or digital communications by nurses trained by the physician and working from established protocols.

Same day acute visits are seen by nurse practitioners or physician assistants working in close collaboration with the physician. The physician's daily work is training and managing the team, as well as seeing the 5-6 patients per day who either require consultation because of the complexity of their disease or who need a procedure. The other 5-6 patients per day are seen for their every 18 month planned visit where their primary care doctor can assist them in mapping out their care for the next 18 months as well as reconnecting on a human level, in a non-rushed visit.

For chronic disease management, groups of patients with the same disease meet with a nurse facilitator in the office in the evening. Their attendance gives them a significant reduction in their co-pay, as well as discounts at local fitness facilities, groceries, and restaurants participating in the wellness plan. Further reductions in co-pays and incentives are provided based on the patient's individual performance with weight, blood pressure, lipids, smoking, and blood sugar control.

Sub-specialty physicians are largely freed from the office and its overhead. They meet with the patient groups with diseases in their specialty area in the medical home and see a few patients individually just after each session there. The bulk of their work day is spent in the hospital performing procedures and managing those with high acuity illness, coordinating care with the primary doctor to keep the length of stay under 3 days.

So, is this view of the future possible? First, will patients be attracted to this model? Early indications are yes, especially the ease of access and the ability to receive care without having to take off work or find child care(2). Is it feasible to make patients more financially accountable for their own health? Robert Brook, one of the most renowned health care researchers at the respected Rand Corporation, makes the case that nothing else will change the behaviors that are draining our health care coffers (3).

Can we really work well in interdisciplinary teams? Those caught up in the battle for and against independent practice for mid-level professionals quote anecdotal information to support their position, but the best scientific study was from the Cochrane Database recently (4). Nurses are good at giving health advice, achieve high levels of patient satisfaction and spend more time with each patient. They may, however, tend to manage complexity and uncertainty by ordering more tests and imaging, inadvertently driving up costs and requiring more invasive testing to chase false positive tests. The ideal situation is a close collaboration where each can function at their best. And we have all known experienced nurses without advanced practice training who are superb in chronic disease management.

Can informatics really help us be better doctors? In my version of 2021, your EHR will have no keyboard. As you sit with your patient at the end of the visit and together review the latest guidelines, your spoken words will become the record of the visit, and the plan will include your patient's words, agreeing to the individual goals for the measures important for his illness. These notes will be for doctors and patients to share, as we're all freed from payment based on how many "bullets" are included or how complex the medical decision-making was. EHR notes will begin to make sense again, and the patient will feel ownership in creating his own story and managing his own health.

Whatever our practice environment in the future, a quote from one of my favorite authors keeps everything in perspective (5). Daniel Sulmasy is a general internist and a Franciscan friar:

The human body is the place where human life and human love happen. The crafts of medicine, nursing, dentistry, and all the other healing arts require at least two human bodies-that of the healer and that of the one who is healed. It is in human bodies that the spirit of God transforms the air we merely breathe into the grace of God that touches every cell in our mortal bodies, forms any words of Good News we will ever proclaim, and moves us to works of charity and worship.

Welcome to my world in 2021. Anybody want to sign up for the voyage? Comments are appreciated at wcrump@trover.org.

## References

1. Greiner AC, Knebel E, Eds: Committee on the Health Professions Education Summit Board on Health Care Services. Health Professions Education: A Bridge to Quality. Washington, DC: Institute of Medicine, National Academy Press; 2003.

2. http://fmignet.aafp.org/online/etc/medialib/fmig

3. Brook RH. Rights and responsibilities in health care. JAMA. 2010;303(22):2289-2290.

4. Laurant M, Reeves D, Hermens R, Braspenning J, et al. Substitution of doctors by nurses in primary care. Cochrane Database of Systematic Reviews 2004, Issue 4. Art No.: CD001271. DOI: 10.1002/14651858.CD001271.pub2.

5. Sulmasy DP. A Balm for Gilead. Washington, D.C. Georgetown University Press. 2006.

*Another inflection point for Dr. Crump was prompted by family illness. His father, previously still vigorous enough to go quail hunting in South Georgia at age 91, was declining and ultimately died after a prolonged hospitalization at age 96. His daughter developed a debilitating chronic disease requiring multiple hospitalizations and only her sheer perseverance got her through medical school. He describes a low point with the image of walking into the local hospital to visit his daughter on the day he should have been across the state at the Academy meeting receiving the teaching faculty of the year award. His cell phone (still a flip phone) rang and his sister in somber tones told him his father might not survive his current hospitalization.*

*After some feelings of hopelessness, he returned to his faith, sacred scripture, and the books recommended years earlier by his daughter. After some time at his father's bedside, he managed to reframe by considering the best of the staff he had encountered in both hospitals. He concluded that the key to healing, especially when cure is not possible, was in embracing the power of hope. He wrote an editorial for each of the journals, knowing they were read by different audiences. He describes writing as therapeutic, and he thought this discovery was too important not to share widely. He has since used the editorials that follow here in every presentation he makes to premedical and preclinical students, and each time he senses their therapeutic value.*

Crump WJ. What Is The Meaning Of Good Doctoring? There Is Hope. Journal of Kentucky Academy of Family Physicians. Fall 2011; 73: 11-13.

**PROLOGUE:** This editorial is written from a distinctly Christian perspective, borrowing widely from Catholic theologians. The tent housing family physicians is large and inclusive, and our Journal welcomes written pieces from all faith traditions and secular perspectives.

I tried several times over the last 4 weeks to sit down and write this editorial. The plan was for me to add another perspective on the family doctor's role in the Patient Centered Medical Home, as so nicely described in other pieces in this issue. I just had to wait until my brain was ready to write, and something entirely unexpected came out.

As I sat with my father during his final illness and death and I continue to stand vigil during my daughter's illness, I encountered many health care workers and physicians in the hospital, doctor's offices, and emergency department. Some knew of my role "behind the curtain" and some did not. Some of them were amazing examples of compassion and caring, and some were not. I wish I could say that compassion tracked with specialty training in our favor, but truthfully some of the best were subspecialists.

As I reflected on this, the concept of "the other," as used in the study of war in history occurred to me (1). Oversimplified, this concept holds that many of man's worst transgressions such as violent racism and brutality in war are explained by the perpetrator truly believing that the victim is so unlike him as to be like a different species. Our interactions with patients are seldom so savage, but the concept is valid, I think.

If I was smart enough to keep quiet, despite pain and nearly complete loss of control, my father and daughter (in hospitalizations separated by space and time) repeatedly connected with their doctors and nurses. I could watch the distance between the patient and the care-giver melt away. Suddenly, instead of "the small bowel obstruction in 368 (the other)," in the eyes of these nurses and doctors, my family became more like their care-givers than different.

I also encountered a few health professionals that never let their guard down. Despite my family's best efforts, the distance never decreased, as they went through the motions of a perfunctory physical exam or charting vital signs and pain scores.

This experience left me entirely unsettled. And when that happens to me, I first turn to Christian Scripture, and then to a favorite book written by a Franciscan friar who is also a general internist (2). And in both sources, there it was, big as life. Some care-givers understand the immense power of hope, and some simply don't.

# FINDING MEANING IN WORK

First, from Hebrews 11:1 with a comment from Sulmasy (2):

"Now faith is being sure of what we hope for and certain of what we do not see."

" Without faith, there can be no hope."

Sebastian Moore wrote that the fundamental question for all humans is whether their life and their person have meaning (3). This passage reads like poetry, and I had to read it twice, slowly, to understand it completely:

"Religion is the believed-in answer of the unknown other, to the question: "Am I valuable in your eyes?" Unless we can come to understand the question as our question and the most human thing about us, we shall never understand the religious answer as the fulfillment of our whole desire for meaning."

So hope is the key, and meaning is the vehicle, as Sulmasy tells us:

"Health care professionals also need to remember that hope is sustained and nurtured in relationship and community. The ultimate end of human hope is a loving relationship with God. But patients can catch glimpses of that ultimate relationship if health care professionals provide them with evidence that they are still very much a part of the human community. People often build walls around the sick. They project onto the sick their own lack of faith, lack of hope, and lack of love. People deny their own death by portraying dying persons as essentially different from them."

Death is not the ultimate enemy- loneliness is. But the physician who provides hope by connecting with the suffering patient and reassuring him that he is valued and really not so much different from the one writing the prescriptions provides a healing force that cannot be matched.

I'll close with a short summary of a talk I gave to the student chapter of the Christian Medical Dental Association at U of L a couple of years ago. Based on Sulmasy's prescription for what he calls the "Prodigal Profession" (2), I suggested a 4-step approach to being the kind of doctor that dispenses hope all day, every day:

1. Every encounter with every patient is an encounter with the mystery of God. He comes to us in the sick, the scarred, and the downcast every day. Strive to experience God's presence at the moment of heal-

ing, and engage each patient with reverent attentiveness. What happens will probably surprise you. Someone from the outside can tell there's something different about your practice.

2. The healer/patient relationship is built on trust. The patient comes to you vulnerable and desperate. Take time to understand these feelings, and act all day, every day like you are worthy of this trust.

3. Keep in mind that the power to heal belongs to God, not you. If you try your best, He'll let you borrow that power from time to time. Every herbal, every pharmaceutical, every machine made of silicon and glass comes to us from Him, so use them wisely.

4. Make a renewed commitment to health care as service. Follow the example of Christ washing the feet of His disciples. And this is not just to recruit more paying patients from your town's best churches to your practice. We serve each patient simply for the sake of serving them, as each is created in the image and likeness of God.

Maybe I did end up writing about the patient centered medical home. We as physicians can't change all the social and financial forces swirling around us. But with the grace of God and a little self-reflection, we can change ourselves. Comments appreciated.

## *References*

1. Clark JA. Unleashing hell: The culture of revenge and the law of retaliation in revolutionary Georgia. Master's Thesis, Eastern Kentucky University. May, 2009.

2. Sulmasy DP. A balm for Gilead. Georgetown University Press. 2006. Washington, DC.

3. Moore S. The fire and the rose are one. Seabury Press. 1980. New York.

# FINDING MEANING IN WORK

Crump WJ. Dispensing Hope: The Fundamental Work of Doctoring. Journal of the Kentucky Medical Association. 2011; 109: 338-339.

**PROLOGUE:** This editorial is written from a distinctly Christian perspective, borrowing widely from Catholic theologians. Portions were previously published in the Journal of the Kentucky Academy of Family Physicians. Our Association is large and inclusive, and our Journal welcomes written pieces from all faith traditions and secular perspectives.

I tried several times over the last 6 weeks to sit down and write this editorial. The plan was for me to add another perspective on the rapid evolution of the Patient Centered Medical Home and newly proposed physician payment mechanisms. I just had to wait until my brain was ready to write, and something entirely unexpected came out.

As I sat with my father during his final illness and death and I continue to stand vigil during my daughter's illness, I encountered many health care workers and physicians in the hospital, doctor's offices, and emergency department. Some knew of my role "behind the curtain" and some did not. Some of them were amazing examples of compassion and caring, and some were not.

As I reflected on this, the concept of "the other," as used in the study of war in history occurred to me (1). Oversimplified, this concept holds that many of man's worst transgressions such as violent racism and brutality in war are explained by the perpetrator truly believing that the victim is so unlike him as to be like a different species. Our interactions with patients are seldom so savage, but the concept is valid, I think.

If I was wise enough to keep quiet, despite pain and nearly complete loss of control, my father and daughter (in hospitalizations separated by space and time) repeatedly connected with their doctors and nurses. I could watch the distance between the patient and the care-giver melt away. Suddenly, instead of "the small bowel obstruction in 368 (the other)," in the eyes of these nurses and doctors, my family became more like their care-givers than different.

I also encountered a few health professionals that never let their guard down. Despite my family's best efforts, the distance never decreased, as they went through the motions of a perfunctory physical exam or charting vital signs and pain scores.

This experience left me entirely unsettled. And when that happens to me, I first turn to Christian Scripture, and then to a favorite book written by a Franciscan friar who is also a general internist (2). And in both sources, there it was, big as life. Some care-givers understand the immense power of hope, and some simply don't.

First, from Hebrews 11:1 with a comment from Sulmasy (2):

"Now faith is being sure of what we hope for and certain of what we do not see."

" Without faith, there can be no hope."

Sebastian Moore wrote that the fundamental question for all humans is whether their life and their person have meaning (3). This passage reads like poetry, and I had to read it twice, slowly, to understand it completely:

"Religion is the believed-in answer of the unknown other, to the question: "Am I valuable in your eyes?" Unless we can come to understand the question as our question and the most human thing about us, we shall never understand the religious answer as the fulfillment of our whole desire for meaning."

So hope is the key, and meaning is the vehicle, as Sulmasy tells us (2):

"Health care professionals also need to remember that hope is sustained and nurtured in relationship and community. The ultimate end of human hope is a loving relationship with God. But patients can catch glimpses of that ultimate relationship if health care professionals provide them with evidence that they are still very much a part of the human community. People often build walls around the sick. They project onto the sick their own lack of faith, lack of hope, and lack of love. People deny their own death by portraying dying persons as essentially different from them."

Death is not the ultimate enemy- loneliness is. But the physician who provides hope by connecting with the suffering patient, reassuring him that he is valued and really not so much different from the one writing the prescriptions, provides a healing force that cannot be matched.

I'll close with a short summary of a talk I gave to the student chapter of the Christian Medical Dental Association at U of L a couple of years ago. Based on Sulmasy's prescription for what he calls the "Prodigal Profession" (2), I suggested a 4-step approach to being the kind of doctor that dispenses hope all day, every day:

1. Every encounter with every patient is an encounter with the mystery of God. He comes to us in the sick, the scarred, and the downcast every day. Strive to experience God's presence at the moment of healing, and engage each patient with reverent attentiveness. What happens will probably surprise you. Someone from the outside can tell there's something different about your practice.

2. The healer/patient relationship is built on trust. The patient comes to you vulnerable and desperate. Take time to understand these feelings, and act all day, every day like you are worthy of this trust.

3. Keep in mind that the power to heal belongs to God, not you. If you try your best, He'll let you borrow that power from time to time. Every herbal, every pharmaceutical, every machine made of silicon and glass comes to us from Him, so use them wisely.

4. Make a renewed commitment to health care as service. Follow the example of Christ washing the feet of His disciples. And this is not just to recruit more paying patients from your town's best churches to your practice. We serve each patient simply for the sake of serving them, as each is created in the image and likeness of God.

Maybe I did end up writing about the patient centered medical home. We as physicians can only do so much to change all the social and financial forces swirling around us. But with the grace of God and a little self-reflection, we can change ourselves. Comments appreciated.

## *References*

1. Clark JA. Unleashing hell: The culture of revenge and the law of retaliation in revolutionary Georgia. Master's Thesis, Eastern Kentucky University. May, 2009.

2. Sulmasy DP. A balm for Gilead. Georgetown University Press. 2006. Washington, DC.

3. Moore S. The fire and the rose are one. Seabury Press. 1980. New York.

### Crump WJ, What Do We Really Know? Some Lessons From Our History. Journal of the Kentucky Medical Association. 2012; (110) 286-288.

As I considered the topic for my editorial this month, I was struck with how history repeats itself, even in medicine. I recently presented one of the series of lectures on medical history that I do every few months for our medical staff, and this time I chose to review childbirth routines in our country since colonial times. When discussing how men midwives entered this picture in the late eighteenth century, we reviewed the standard treatments of the time for difficult labor and for pain relief.

In 1810, a physician writer suggested bleeding the patient who had a slow labor to the point of fainting, often followed (by his report) of improved results (1). The Chamberlen family's well-kept secret for almost 3 generations ultimately brought forceps delivery into vogue. Although these instruments were undoubtedly valuable in selected cases in well-trained hands, their use by inexperienced "regular doctors" trained only by apprenticeship caused severe lacerations leading to death or permanent fistulas (2, 3). The pressure to "just do something" was just too great for these inexperienced birth attendants to let nature take its course, even if slowly.

The most common medicinal pain relief of the time was laudanum, an alcohol based tincture of opium. It was probably effective, but also contained narcotine, a powerful emetic. The laboring woman traded less pain for more vomiting. Later in the nineteenth century, the discovery of ether brought real pain relief to the bedside. Followed by the development of chloroform and nitrous oxide, these agents were initially used lightly so that in 1880, 50% of deliveries used anesthesia but only 8% required forceps (3). Later, deeper levels were used without any control of the airway, with the result that the maternal mortality rate persisted at almost 50 per 10,000, nearly 25 times the number we see today. This prompted the New York Health Commissioner to say in 1934: "I have seen hundreds of women die on the delivery table because of the wrongful use of these drugs."(3).

A closer look at the maternal mortality rate in 1880 that had not changed since the 1700s revealed that infection in the form of childbed fever was a large factor. While most physicians have heard the Semmelweis story from 1846, this disease was actually well-described in 1746 by Paul Malouin at the Hotel Dieu in Paris. A classic example of seeing what you look for, he described the autopsy findings of diffuse peritoneal exudate as curdled milk. This image of obstructed milk causing life threatening fever so captivated the anatomists of the day that there were drawings of a (non-existent) duct connecting the breast with the uterus. Alexander Gordon in Aberdeen in 1780 recognized the temporal correlation between puerperal fever and skin infections, and suggested transmissibility: "The disease seized such women only as were visited, or delivered by a practitioner…who has previously attended patients with the disease. It is a disagreeable declaration for me to mention that I was myself the means of carrying the infection to a great number of women." (1).

Although not published until 1846, Semmelweis recognized in the early 1800s that those women attended in the physician- managed first division of the Vienna Lying In Hospital had almost double the rate of mortality of the second division which was managed by midwives. Careful review showed that the medical students examining laboring patients in the first division began their day in the morgue, dissecting corpses of women who had died recently. They went directly from this activity to the labor wards without washing their hands. The familiar version of the story concludes with enforced hand-washing with chlorinated lime resulting in a dramatic decrease in maternal mortality. While this is true, there was a very long delay between recognition by visionaries and the application by the medical students and their faculty. This delay was caused by what they thought they knew and their stubborn unwillingness to consider the facts.

This inability to recognize the true cause of many infections was a key factor in President Garfield's death in 1880. Detailed in a fascinating recent book I recommend to anyone with an interest in medical history, it was not the assassin's bullet that killed him (4). Despite the wide acceptance of the need for antisepsis in Europe following Lister's publications in the 1860s, American physicians considered it ridiculous. The result was that the best physicians and surgeons in America were called to the fallen president's bedside. They repeatedly probed, with unwashed bare hands and unsterilized instruments, the presumed path of the bullet. Because of what they thought they knew: the bullet must be removed. This was despite many reports of Civil War wounded who walked around quite well with fragments of lead bullets in various body cavities.

The drama was heightened when Alexander Graham Bell, the noted inventor, was called to the president's bedside to attempt to locate the bullet with his newest invention. This induction coil, an early metal detector, let the entire country down when it could not locate the bullet. Only when the president died a slow septic death 11 weeks after being shot and an autopsy was done did the extent of what they didn't know become obvious. The bullet had passed from the right side of the lower back, through a vertebral body, missed all vessels and nerves, and lodged harmlessly behind the pancreas on the left, just adjacent to the hilum of the spleen. The tract on the right that had been developed from the entry wound was enlarged and infected from repeated procedures by those who thought they knew what to do. And the chief physician, Dr. D. Willard Bliss, was so certain of the location of the bullet in that track that he had confined Bell's search to the right side. Later, Bell's invention would prove effective in other gunshot victims.

So the president's doctors, and not the assassin, had killed him. How could they have been so wrong? When Lister's process of using carbolic acid to dress wounds and provide antisepsis was brought to America and promoted by Oliver Wendell Holmes, Sr, in 1842, he was derided publicly. The Editor of a highly respected American journal of the time said: "…we are likely to be as much ridiculed in the next century for our blind belief in the power of unseen germs, as our forefathers were for their faith in the influence of spirits…"

One of President Garfield's attending physicians, after the autopsy was complete, said simply: "…We made a mistake." A famous German surgeon of the time summarized the key issue: "It seems that the attending physicians were under the pressure of the public opinion that they were doing far too little. But according to my opinion they have done…too much."

History's lessons are here today to be learned. A recent report noted that as much as 30% of the cost of American health care is spent on services that provide no real benefit to the patient (5). A recent multispecialty panel report made the bold recommendation that we stop doing some routine things that have no evidence to support them (6). Will we change from what we think we know? Sometimes the more we really know, the less we should do. Listening carefully to the patient's story, providing some relief of their distress, and nurturing hope for their future may be the most valuable thing we can do.

## *References*

1. Loudon I. Western medicine. Oxford: Oxford University Press. 1997.
2. Leavitt JW. Science enters the birthing room. The Journal of American History. 1983; 70 (2): 281-304.
3. Borst CG. Catching Babies. Cambridge: Harvard University Press. 1995
4. Millard C. Destiny of the republic: A tale of madness, medicine, and the murder of a president. New York: Doubleday. 2011
5. Garber A, Goldman DP, Jena AB. The promise of health care cost containment. Health Aff (Millwood). 2007;26(6):1545-1547.
6. http://choosingwisely.org/, accessed May 30, 2012.

**Crump WJ. Time to Remove the Pump Handle? Lessons for the Provision of Modern Medical Care from Dr. John Snow and the Broad Street Pump. Journal of the Kentucky Medical Association. 2013; (111): 134-136.**

By the time this editorial is published, I will have been to my first Bob Dylan concert. Despite having been drawn to his lyrics and music for as long as I can remember, our paths just haven't crossed. Aficionados like me will remember the line "The pump don't work 'Cause the vandals took the handles" from his Subterranean Homesick Blues. This confluence occurs within weeks of the 200th anniversary of the birthday of John Snow, the father of modern epidemiology. Many will remember the story.

After an apprenticeship with a surgeon in Newcastle-upon-Tyne, Snow got his first view of cholera when he was 18. At age 23, he moved to London, finished his medical training, and at age 32 established practice in Soho, a gritty working class neighborhood (1).

Londoners in 1848 shared their living space with a menagerie of horses and livestock, and sewage either accumulated in the streets or found its way directly into the Thames River. Waves of cholera would take their toll, and before the discovery of microbial pathogenesis, the most common hypothesis for its cause was the Hippocratic concept of Miasma (Greek for pollution). In this belief system, the toxic agent was thought to contaminate inhaled air, which then upset the person's balance of the four humors, allowing yellow bile (choler) to accumulate, requiring the body to expel it exuberantly, often resulting in massive dehydration and sometimes death.

Using his earlier work with ether and chloroform, Snow questioned the common understanding. If Miasma were the culprit, why were the garbage collectors and "night-soil men" who emptied the outhouses not at increased risk? And how could the gas reach an entire sprawling city? By "gumshoe" epidemiology, he carefully studied everything about each cholera case, including their water bills that cited the source of the water. In his own area of Soho, he tracked the 500 cases back to a single public water source near a contaminated house, the Broad Street pump. Once he convinced the local leaders to remove the pump handle making it inaccessible, the rate of cholera dropped dramatically. The rest, as they say, is history. Hand washing, aggressively washing dirty linens, and boiling all water sources became the life-saving technology of the day. It would be 35 years later that Robert Koch and Louis Pasteur identified Vibrio cholera in Egypt, vindicating Snow 25 years after his death of a cerebral hemorrhage.

Londoners in Snow's time couldn't help themselves. Despite disease, death, and filth all around them, water was basic to life. Physicians of the time also couldn't see "the forest for the trees," busily treating the sad cases that presented on their doorstep, believing the science of the day, and not worrying much about what was happening on Broad Street. A series of recent editorials has suggested that now is the time to use the concepts of public health to solve the major threats of our day: How do we get affordable health care to those who need it without endangering our financial ability to provide the other basics of a modern society like security and education? And how do we address the epidemic of chronic disease driven by lifestyle choices such as obesity and smoking?

Beginning with the first question, the key word is the NEEDED health care. Recent studies have shown that fully 30% of the care we provide, including some very expensive tests and interventions, do not benefit our patients (2). In fact, because of false-positive findings generating follow-up tests and procedures that result in complications, we may actually be harming our patients. But we can't help ourselves. Patients present on our doorstep with complaints that COULD be caused by something scary, and they expect us to use all modern technology to address their (and our) unease with anything but complete knowledge of their bodily functions. Even as we work away, pumping as fast as we can, many of us suspect that maybe we're on the wrong track. But we may get sued if we don't keep pumping, and everything in our culture rewards doing more, even if it breaks the bank.

So how can we do less? A particularly brave report from the American Board of Internal Medicine Foundation recently clearly recommended that many common protocols of evaluation and treatment are not supported by good evidence, and should be excluded from our routines (3). Over 35 other specialty societies have now joined this effort, adding their lists. A less helpful way of addressing this issue is the phrase "waste, abuse, and fraud" sometimes included under the less offensive rubric of "program integrity" (4). Those of us who toil in the trenches know that there is very little conscious self-aggrandizing "fraud" by physicians, but on reflection, most will admit that the momentum to do more testing and treatment is sometimes hard to resist.

One method to do less is to align profit with patient outcomes. The concept of Accountable Care Organizations (ACOs) included in the Affordable Care act (ACA) seems to be here to stay, after the recent Supreme Court decision. More than just the old-fashioned Health Maintenance Organizations (HMOs) and capitation systems of the 1990s, the ACO has similar goals: control costs, facilitate quality, and improve population health. What's different is that all services needed are to be included in a global payment to the entity that accepts responsibility for a defined population of patients. So this includes not only inpatient and outpatient medical care, but home health, nursing home care, durable equipment, and pharmacy. Much like Diagnosis Related Groups (DRGs) transformed inpatient care from a slow, per-diem driven "pump" to a (mostly) efficient assembly line, ACOs have the potential to streamline the process, but are more comprehensive. This is a sea change. The ACO that finds and excludes the 30% of care that doesn't help our patients will be extremely profitable, while those who continue "business as usual" won't last long.

This is scary. When an endoscopy unit or catheterization lab suddenly moves from being considered a revenue center to a cost center, the ground starts shaking. Which CTs and MRIs in the ED are really needed? Just asking the question is threatening to the makers of the machines and those who chose a specialty based on our current high utilization rates. Will someone have the gumption to remove the pump handle? Even more problematic, as currently envisioned, the John Snows of our time won't have the authority or motivation. Two recent editorials have noted that ACOs as currently framed really accept the responsibility only for the medical care of their covered lives, not the true population health (5,6). If health were really the goal, resources would be invested in the real social causes of many of our chronic diseases. Causes sometimes associated with the left side of the political spectrum like addressing issues with housing, education, poverty, and nutrition and a team that truly integrates empowered social services providers would be an integral part of HEALTH care. Does that sound too much like Miasma to us?

I'll close with a couple of stories, perhaps apocryphal, that underline the importance of doing less in this brave new world. The first comes from my time as the medical monitor for Space Station design in the 90s. NASA focused much effort on the concept of "human factors" that could make or break an otherwise ideal engineering design. The story is told that several companies were vying to take over the hearing aid market by making smaller, less noticeable in-the-ear devices. Vexed by the inability to find the design they sought, they contracted with NASA Research and Development folks. It only took a few months for them to discern that there was a size, shape, and color that optimized effectiveness and anything smaller just wouldn't work as well. Nothing in the physics of sound transmission explained this threshold. It was the human factors folks who solved the puzzle. If the device was too small to be seen easily by those speaking to the wearer, the speaker didn't raise their voice enough to be heard easily.

The second is from the North Carolina Medicaid system that has functioned as a type of ACO for several years, saving the state almost $300 million dollars so far. The funds are allocated to a community-driven Board that is responsible for a natural service area of 3-5 counties rather than by a bureaucrat hundreds of miles away. It is up to that Board to decide how to spend the money. The story is told that there was this one elderly woman who lived out in the county, about 30 miles from the nearest hospital. Her anxiety would get out of control, she would begin having chest pain, and call EMS to take her to the hospital. Never knowing how long it would take them to arrive, she worried more and more. By the time she got to the ED the picture was very impressive. After 5 such visits and admissions, the medical staff thought that a negative cardiac cath would reassure her. It did not. The cycle continued. On the advice of her physician, the Board made a bold move. They took Medicaid funds and rented an apartment for her across the street from the ED, where staff could walk over and see her as needed. The cycle was broken, and thousands of dollars were saved.

Where are our John Snows? Who is bold enough to remove the pump handle? Comments appreciated.

## *References*

1. Markel H. Happy birthday, Dr. Snow. JAMA. 2013;309 (5):995-996.

2. Berwick DM, Hackbarth AD. Eliminating waste in US health care. JAMA. 2012;307(14): 1513-1516.

3. http://www.choosingwisely.org/. Accessed April 11, 2013.

4. Agrawal S, Taitsman J, Cassel C. Educating physicians about responsible management of finite resources. JAMA. 2013;309(11): 1115-1116

5. Noble DJ, Casalino LP. Can accountable care organizations improve population health? Should they try? JAMA. 2013;309(11): 1119-1120.

6. Shortell SM. Bridging the divide between health and health care. JAMA. 2013;309(11): 1121-1122.

## Crump WJ. Tending the Medical Home: 2013. Journal of the Kentucky Academy of Family Physicians. Summer 2013; (79): 11-14.

The process of providing health care in this country is broken. This is not news to anyone who has tried to be there for their patients while still paying the bills. A system "designed" to meet the needs of acute illnesses paid for out of pocket (or with a barter system using vegetables and fowl) by the patient worked fairly well in the 1910s. Doctors provided "charity care" because it was the right thing to do, and there was enough profit in the overall system to support this approach. Then insurance companies stepped in to lessen the short-term financial impact on the individual patient. For catastrophic costs, this system seemed to make sense. For day-to-day care, it obviously benefited the insurers, who made money, invested it, and made more money. Fee-for-service including insurance payments was still profitable for doctors and hospitals, despite an entire new layer of necessary billing and the wasted effort involved. Each patient had a personal family doctor, subspecialists were rare, and costs were reasonable.

There is no agreement on when this changed, but most cite the advent of Medicare in 1965, followed by Medicaid. For a while, it seemed to make sense. Medicare provided health insurance for those 65 years old and older and the disabled. Medicaid covered the poor who were also in a vulnerable situation, such as pregnant patients and children. Doctors and hospitals were paid a reasonable rate, elders could spend less time worrying about financial ruin caused by a prolonged illness, and Medicaid payment for charity care at least covered the overhead costs, if not compensating for the doctors' time. Medicaid coverage for obstetrical care provided more accessible prenatal care and delivery, and children of poor families could get preventive and illness care.

Then something happened. Medical care became a commodity, and a fashionable one at that. Americans saw the medical system as another place to shop for the best, and the solid American concept of "more must be best" flourished. At the same time, subspecialties were born. Even at this point, most of a person's care was provided or closely managed by their personal physician. Family Medicine became a Board certified specialty in 1969. Then the next big thing happened. Medical technology exploded. The diagnostician's hands, eyes, and ears were largely replaced with elegant imaging capabilities. Fiber optic and then digital cameras were made so small and reliable that there was almost no internal structure that couldn't be accessed from some orifice. Subspecialists could focus on "their" orifice or "oscopy" and became "ologists." A very large, expensive but still profitable industry was developed that grew more rapidly than automotive manufacturing, the previous leader, and made the U.S. the envy of the world. Especially in our cities, an individual's prestige was marked by how many subspecialists he had seen and how many orifices had been traversed.

Then we realized that we couldn't afford this monster that we had built. Patients were only paying 10-20% of the real cost of each ologist expedition, and the poor were paying nothing. Our government, knowing that Americans would never voluntarily give up such a good deal, tightened the screws on doctors and hospitals. Generous per diem rates to hospitals changed to a prospective payment system for DRGs. This meant that the hospital was paid a flat rate by severity of illness of their patient, no matter how long the patient stayed in the hospital. Overnight, the usual profit margin of 15-20% dropped dramatically. A good small business might have a profit margin of 10%. Hospitals now were functioning at the 1-3% level.

It was harder for the payers to cut doctors' payments. There is serious talk now about paying doctors by a fixed payment per ambulatory episode of care, but the real cost is still the fees for procedures, emergency department visits, and hospitalization. The government has just taken the "slow drain" approach. By failing to increase payments to doctors to keep up with inflation, they are effectively paying them less each year. With the advent of Accountable Care Organizations, the government is hoping that costs can be controlled by putting doctors and hospitals at risk in the same financial entity.

But where were our patients during all this upheaval? Most continued on their usual way, dining from the ologist menu as needed. In the late 1980s, led by an upstart group of academic family doctors, the negatives of this approach for patients became apparent. False positive tests led to more tests, sometimes biopsies, and some patients were harmed. Medicines were not without side effects, and hospitals could be dangerous places. Seeing several different doctors at the same time led to hazardous overlaps in treatments and emergency departments often repeated unnecessary tests, with more false positives, and the cycle continued. The value of continuity of care was clear to our patients, we thought.

The failure of the health care reforms of the Clinton era can be blamed on many things, but many believe it was largely because the American public simply was not ready to be constrained by a "gatekeeper" standing between them and the ologist menu. Most saw this as just a way to keep them from spending "their money" that the insurance companies or the government owed them. Americans did not understand, or believe in, the concept that a personal physician coordinating their care would not only save money but was actually better for them as individuals.

So what's different now? We have 20 years more data from leaders like Dr. Barbara Starfield and others that make the case even more strongly. Many more specialty societies have publicly supported the concept of the Patient Centered Medical Home (PCMH). Fortune 500 companies are "all in" on the concept. Demonstration projects with federal funding are underway to pay primary care physicians for managing patients over time whether they are seen in the office or not. For the first time in almost 100 years, primary care physicians may be paid what they are truly worth again. But the determining factor on whether the current PCMH movement will succeed or go the way of the Clinton health plan will be the attention paid to the first two words of the new effort. What makes what we do PATIENT CENTERED?

In the editorial I wrote in this journal in 2007 on this issue (1), I summarized a 2006 piece (2) that still provides a nice framework for our current efforts. In the other articles in this issue of your journal, we will showcase some current efforts in our state. As you read them, consider how each approaches the following 4 questions:

How does this effort:

1. Make it easier for patients to get access to care and obtain continuity

2. Provide ways to increase the patient's participation in their care

3. Provide the skills necessary for patient self-care

4. Coordinate care among different clinical settings?

We hope to provide summaries of how our membership is addressing these important questions along with updates on those leading the effort in future issues. We invite you to send us summaries of your efforts. Let's get this right this time. The stakes are just too high to let others mandate where and how we do this doctoring thing.

## *References*

1. Crump WJ. What if family doctors were paid for tending the medical home? J Ky Acad Fam Physicians 2007; 57: 3-5.

2. Bergeson SC, Dean JD. A systems approach to patient-centered care. JAMA 2006;296:2848-51.

## Crump, WJ. Consensus Guidelines or Clinical Jazz: How Should Our Care Be Measured? Journal of the Kentucky Medical Association. 2014; (112): 78-80.

As I considered a useful topic for this month's editorial, I had an interesting confluence of events in one day. In my role as Dean of a regional campus and teacher of medical students, I review all the care we provide in our student-led free clinic. Each new Class of M-3s reviews the chronic care protocols from the class just previous and decides how they should be changed. Then we review the charts as a group and provide feedback to each other as to how well we've followed our protocols and how to work in a truly collaborative fashion with our patients. As I often remind the students, it's the patient's diabetes (hypertension, dyslipidemia, COPD, etc.), not yours. If we try to "walk a mile in their shoes," we are more likely to understand how best to work our suggestions into our patients' everyday lives, with better long term results.

Although new evidence is published all the time, we don't have to change the protocols too much. For instance, when the ACCOMPLISH trial (1) showed that calcium channel blockers were superior to other second choice medications for hypertension in most patients, it required little modification of our routines, as we weren't prescribing many beta blockers or hydrochlorothiazide anyway. The consensus panel statement on dyslipidemia was 13 years old and the one for hypertension was 11 years old, but no new national guidelines had been published. This meant that what we did in free clinic was the same as what were considered the "right answers" to the questions on the students' exams that were written probably several years ago. This was a great longitudinal way to reinforce what they were learning on their block rotations, and our students did well.

Within the space of 2 months, our comfortable world of guidelines changed. New lipid guidelines were released, and I guess it's revealing that I first heard about this on a radio news program. "Millions more will now be prescribed statins" was the headline. This is a really interesting story, as most of the suggested guidelines had been ready for 6-8 years, but the key authors couldn't agree on some of the details, and the sponsoring entity finally gave up and got out of the guideline business. This left the American College of Cardiology/American Heart Association to take over publication of the guidelines. Reluctantly, I obtained the publication and worked my way through an obtuse review of the new evidence (2). I was heartened to see that one thing I had taught my students for years was corroborated. There never was much evidence that the non-statin lipid drugs were effective, and prescribing them and their side effects to asymptomatic patients has never made sense to me. The guideline made that case. And they made the case that I have also taught for years that only LDL cholesterol reliably predicted vascular disease and any other sub fractions were unnecessary.

But wait, they were also saying that the tried and true method of setting an LDL goal based on risk factors and then titrating the statin dose was passé. They said that the evidence doesn't support this and now we should only use those risks to determine which intensity statin to use, prescribe it at a fixed dose, and then only check LDL periodically to assess for compliance. I don't like this anymore than I like not checking a PTT when prescribing low molecular weight heparin, but I got accustomed to that so surely I could learn this too. But then they offended my baby boomer sensibilities even further by suggesting that the decision to treat asymptomatic patients should be based on a calculation that I couldn't do in my head. In fact, I now needed to use an on-line calculator to estimate if my patient's risk exceeded the magic number. Or, I could get this calculator as an "app" for my phone. I looked down at my belt at the last remaining flip phone among our faculty, and finally gave in and got a smart phone. That really hurt – a phone that is smarter than I am.

And then the JNC 8 hypertension guidelines were published (3). And here were some more blockbuster suggestions. First, they tell us that there's no evidence to treat patients with known vascular or kidney disease or diabetes to a lower blood pressure, saying 140/90 is good enough. As this heresy settled in, I could hear a distant rumble of the organizations advocating for those diseases assembling their forces to battle this new guideline. And then they said that those 60 and older should be considered controlled at anything below 150/90. At first this seemed to support my bias that tight control of blood pressure in the elderly often caused more broken hips than saved heart attacks. But wait, this new guideline would apply to me, and I'm certainly not elderly- Am I?

Already there has been a flurry of editorials questioning the wisdom of these two new guidelines (4-6). The point is made that most of the individuals who would volunteer their time over many years to work on these guidelines had close ties to the pharmaceutical corporations. Others, while free of this bias, are leaders of subspecialty clinical enterprises that would greatly benefit from more aggressive management of asymptomatic patients with these conditions. So what do I tell my students?

For a while, this answer isn't too hard. Since the right answers on their tests won't change for several years, I could stall, just going with business as usual. I explained the rationale behind the new guidelines and prepared them for the controversy they might hear from their subspecialty faculty, but our protocols are safe for now. But then that same day I was seeing patients in my office and I was staring right into the horns of the dilemma.

My first patient was a 56 year old marginally controlled type 2 diabetic who also had hypertension. As the evidence accumulated that tight control of blood sugar actually might increase cardiovascular mortality in these patients, I had already begun to be satisfied with a higher hemoglobin A1C. In fact, I had adopted the "hand" approach to managing these patients (7). Based on the evidence, this approach says that control of blood sugar with insulin is the least important aspect of caring for type 2 diabetics, while smoking cessation, BP control, metformin therapy, and lipid control are the most important. But her BP had been in the range of 135/85 over the last three visits, and her ACE and HCTZ were maxed out. Based on the old guidelines, I needed to add a calcium channel blocker. Based on the new guidelines, things were just fine. What's a good doctor to do?

My next patient was a 62 year old with mild hypertension and recently diagnosed dyslipidemia. We were in the process of titrating his statin upward to the goal based on the previous guideline, using a low potency statin because his co-pay for it was the least. But the new guideline (and the "app" that I resent), says I should use a high potency statin and not bother with following the LDL. What would Marcus Welby do?

In both situations, two quotes from my former mentors at Vandy and UAB popped into my head. First, "when there's more than one right option, let the patient choose their poison." Next, "the mark of a good clinician is to know when not to follow the guidelines." Then I considered one of my favorite concepts, that of "clinical jazz"(8). In jazz, that most American form of art, the printed score is just a suggestion, with improvisation seen as the highest accomplishment. And so the published guideline is the equivalent of the score, and providing some "off guideline" care might just be in order. So, as best I could, I explained to these patients our options and what we think we know (today) about each, and guided them to make their own decisions. The first chose the more aggressive option for BP control, and the other chose just to continue the low co-pay statin. And I left my office that day feeling that I had been a good doctor.

But all is not well in the clinical guideline world. As discussed in the editorials referenced above, guidelines have a way of creeping into standards by which our care is measured. On my most cynical of days I envision someone with a high school education and the old Type 2 diabetes guidelines finding my patient's A1C of 7.1% "below standards" and refusing to put a smiley face on my report card. Even worse, in the near future this "below standard" care might result in a significant financial penalty both to me and my group. How can I possibly explain clinical jazz to bean counters?

And what do I tell my students that won't make them more cynical than they already are? I always fall back on a basic cross cultural explanation (9). After considerable study, Howard Brody summarized that in all cultures around the world, healers do basically three things:

1. Provide a meaningful explanation for the illness

2. Express care and concern

3. Manage the possibility of mastery and control over the illness or its symptoms

One of the descriptions of the derivation of the word guidelines comes from snow skiing. Here, the experienced guide sets up ropes to keep the skier in the safe area. So, the question becomes, who is the best guide for our patients: an expert who has spent much time lost in the snow or the less experienced guide who knows well the strengths and weaknesses of the skier being guided?

In my world view faith is an important part of this effort, and not knowing our patients' faith tradition would be like not knowing their BP or LDL. So by truly understanding our patients, choosing the "right thing" seems to come easier. And with some prayer and a bit of reflection, I can face whatever the guideline forces of darkness have in store for me.

Comments appreciated.

## *References*

1. Jamerson KA, Bakris GL, Wun CC, et al. Rationale and design of the avoiding cardiovascular events through combination therapy in

patients living with systolic hypertension (ACCOMPLISH) trial: the first randomized controlled trial to compare the clinical outcome effects of first-line combination therapies in hypertension. Am J Hypertens 2004; 17:793.

2. Stone NJ, Robinson J, Lichtenstein AH, et al.ACC/AHA Guideline on the Treatment of Blood Cholesterol to Reduce Atherosclerotic Cardiovascular Risk in Adults: a report of the American College of Cardiology/American Heart Association Task Force on Practice Guidelines [published online November 12, 2013]. Circulation. doi:10.1161/01.cir.0000437738.63853.7a.

3. James PA, Oparil S, Carter BL, et al. 2014 Evidence-based guidelines for management of high blood pressure in adults. Report from the panel members appointed to the eighth joint national committee (JNC 8). JAMA 2014;311(5):507-520.

4. 4) Ioannidis JPA. More than a billion people taking statins? Potential implications of the new cardiovascular guidelines. JAMA 2014;311(5):463-464.Montori VM, Brito JP, Ting HH. Patient-centered and practical application of new high cholesterol guidelines to prevent cardiovascular disease. JAMA 2014;311(5):465-466.

5. Freiden TR, King SMC, Wright JS. Protocol-based treatment of hypertension. A critical step on the pathway to progress. JAMA 2014;311(1):21-22.

6. Erlich DR, Slawson DC, Shaughnessy AF. "Lending a Hand" to patients with type 2 diabetes: A simple way to communicate treatment goals. Am Fam Phys 2014;89(4):256-258.

7. Shaughnessy AF, Slawson DC, Becker L. Clinical jazz: Harmonizing clinical experience and evidence-based medicine. J Fam Pract. 1998 Dec;47(6):425-8.Borkan J, Reis S, Steinmetz D, and Medalie JH. Patients and Doctors. Life changing stories from primary care. The University of Wisconsin Press. Madison, WI. 1999.

**Crump WJ. Genomics, Personalized Medicine, and Population Health: Who really needs a family doctor? Kentucky Academy of Family Physicians. Winter 2015; (83): 18-20.**

The appearance of the first few words of the title in a recent editorial caught my attention, hoping that some esteemed cardiologists at a big name institution had finally tumbled to the importance of what we family docs do every day (1). Before I share my disappointment, a couple of cases from my own recent experience:

JW is a 48 year old woman who I have seen over the last 10 years with mixed anxiety and depression who generally presents with a somatic complaint that is easily evaluated, treated, and reassurance is appreciated. The time she had an unusual breast calcification was a bit more stressful for us both, but a close personal relationship I had with a good surgeon resulted in a very quick and reassuring biopsy.

This time she complained of back pain at work and was referred to the occupational medicine physician under worker's compensation. A few days after her outpatient consultation with him, she was on my schedule for an urgent evaluation. She described the pain as radiating down her left leg and leaving a "funny" pain/numbness in her foot. He did some x-rays and she heard him say that he was concerned it might be an aortic aneurysm or something like multiple sclerosis. He advised a CT scan and neurologist consultation. She was, quite simply, terrified. She had not been able to sleep and was afraid to work, and had been just staying at home.

Her exam showed a classic positive straight-leg raise and bow string test on the left, decreased sensation in the L-4/L-5 distribution, normal strength throughout, and no other neurological findings. Her pulses were excellent in both lower extremities and had normal capillary refill. Reflecting on her history, I had helped her quit smoking 8 years ago, she had a low LDL cholesterol, no diabetes, and an unremarkable family history. I told her it seemed like a small "slipped disc" to me, and left the room to review her films.

Her films were done at another facility, so I didn't have access. When I returned to the room and told her this, one could observe her become more tense. "What should I do?" she said with a quivering voice. I told her that if I were her, I'd take the NSAID that we've used before for musculoskeletal pain, return to the Occ med doc as planned in two days and ask him to call me while she was there, and stop worrying. She agreed to do all but the latter. I made a mental note to consider adding gabapentin later if the NSAID didn't allow her to work.

The call didn't come, and I assumed things must have settled down because I didn't hear from her as I usually would. About a week later I got a 20 page fax from a physician group I didn't recognize that included a neurologist note complete with NCV and EMG, CT and MRI that showed a mild L-4/5 radiculopathy with a bulging disc at that level. He had also done a huge lab evaluation for vasculitis and connective tissue disease that showed only a minimally elevated RA titer with a low sedimentation rate that generally means nothing. He made an appointment for her with a rheumatologist.

So she came to me again, distraught (the last thing she heard was "could be rheumatoid arthritis"), and the pain was no better. She now had an appointment with a spine surgeon and a rheumatologist and had seen plenty of on-line photos of "crippling RA." Again, "what should I do?" I told her I thought in her situation the RA titer was a false positive and suggested we start a trial of increasing doses of gabapentin. Once we saw how much she could do at work and home, she would be ready to discuss options with the spine surgeon.

On her way out, she said "you made me feel SO much better," and she was optimistic again. I thought to myself, "Well, I guess that's my job." I also had to shake my head, knowing that our health system would pay our office about 5% of the total cost of her evaluation by others for my simple history, physical, assessment, and plan.

The next was an OB patient:

SR is 19 years old, pregnant with her first child at about 18 weeks. Just as we were about to load up and leave our prenatal clinic that is 45 minutes way from Madisonville where we needed to be at noon conference in an hour, our receptionist called me and said SR had just arrived, an hour late for her appointment. Knowing that it's often difficult for SR to get away from her job on time, I could sense our receptionist's disapproval as I said

# FINDING MEANING IN WORK

that we would see her. And the look on our nurse's face was even more expressive. She set all of our portable office back down, and brought SR back to be seen.

As I entered some notes, the PG-2 resident saw her first as we usually do. I could hear the Doppler crackling and whining with occasional static but not the regular "baby music" that is a good, loud, reassuring fetal heartbeat (FHTs). I looked up to see our nurse joining him in the exam room with another Doppler, also followed only by noise. Thoughts raced in my head. We had heard the FHTs last visit, and an ultrasound 2 weeks ago confirmed her dates.

As I considered the worst, images of the three generations of this family that I know came to mind. And how this young woman, the oldest in her generation, was clearly the shining star. She had done well in school, followed all the rules (and this family has a bunch of rules) and married well. This pregnancy was carefully planned to allow her to continue community college on time so she could begin nursing school while her extended family provided the best day care. How was I going to tell her if the news was bad?

I had struggled with these antiquated Dopplers for 10 years, and knew they each had loose wires that had to be coddled just right to make a good connection. I conjured up all of my professional demeanor and entered the exam room with a reassuring smile on my face. She was supine on the table staring at the ceiling with both hands white-knuckled on the sides of the exam table. Both resident and nurse looked as if they'd rather be anywhere but here. I added much more gel to her belly, took the better of the two Dopplers, asked the resident to hold one of the connections tightly, and proceed to search for this 2 centimeter flickering heart. Thankfully, we found it quickly and the rhythmic beat filled the room.

One could watch everyone in the room relax, and she looked at me and said, almost inaudibly, "thank you, I feel so much better now." My heart rate was still too close to that of the fetus to think it then, but later, again, "Well, I guess that's my job." I also could very clearly remember that in that same room 6 years ago the outcome was not so good. "Thank you, God."

So why was I so disappointed in the editorial from the cardiologists? Their extolling the benefits of population health started out well, as I agreed that we are responsible for the patients in our practice whether we see them or not. In fact, one of the key strategies of the Patient Centered Medical Home (PCMH) for which I routinely advocate is the ability to manage our patients actively between office visits. I was disappointed because their view of population health was studying "big data" from electronic health records (EHR) to find the folks who have the disease that belongs to each "ologist" and then studying outcomes of various interventions on that population. As I stared at the barely intelligible notes that our EHR created for me on these two patients, I couldn't find anything describing the importance of what happened. In fact, as I discuss EHR templates with family docs around the country, they decry the loss of nearly everything important that happens in an office visit, hidden by the haze of useless details.

Well, at least I could agree with the editorialists about personalized medicine, right? Disappointed again. This term to them meant knowing the genetic markers of a cancer to choose the best chemotherapy or the precise hepatitis C genotype to choose treatment. This aspect of genomics is in its infancy, but soon knowing the patient's molecular make-up will really help with choice of treatment of more diseases. Anybody who has been in practice for a while has seen that a medication that works in one member of a family is often the best first choice for other relatives.

So what do we family docs mean by personalized medicine? To me, it is the realization that precious few illnesses are truly cured, and that the somatic symptoms for which regular folks seek medical attention require a healing force that can't be pressed into a pill. What most patients seek is careful listening by a trusted doctor, a physical exam with the therapeutic effect of touch, and then reassurance and symptomatic treatment with few side effects. But they also trust us to find the "zebras among the horses" that do require further testing and consultation. The dance that results is best done to a score written by the relationship between the healer and the healed. This is personalized care, and cannot be provided by a stranger.

A book I've recommended before in these pages is Jack Medalie et al's Life-changing stories from primary care (2). In the introduction to the section on Family and Community, Howard Brody fleshes out this concept of relationship-centered care

"To be human is to be shaped inevitably by one's culture, but to be shaped in a way which is simultaneously and constantly influenced by our family background and by our own individual personality. No two people are members of a culture in quite the same way; simply knowing a list of cultural beliefs and practices is insufficient to understand how any individual within that culture will behave or what he or she will value."

Brody goes on to summarize the 3 essential elements common to all healing practices in all cultures:

1. Provide a meaningful explanation for the illness

2. Express care and concern

3. Manage the possibility of mastery and control over the illness or its symptoms

Good doctoring means accomplishing those three tasks and this is impossible without solid, trusting relationships. Philip Yancy, in his delightful treatise on the Christian concept of grace (another book I strongly recommend), reviews the sociologic concept of the looking-glass self (3). This view holds that you become what the most influential people in your life think you are. Could it be that our relationships with our patients actually define who we are as doctors?

And Brody again:

"The centrality of relationship as a way of both knowing and healing in primary care brings us back again to the importance of local knowledge. One forms relationships not with abstractions, but with specific people, families, and communities. ... even caring physicians dedicated to these relationships may fail, but physicians neglectful or dismissive of these relationships will almost certainly fail." Is it any wonder that our current medical system in America fails so many of us?

So I'm not sure exactly how or why I made these patients feel better, but I know it has something to do with our relationship. So in this brave new world of "big data," genomics, and modern population medicine, who needs a family doctor?

We all do. Comments appreciated.

## References

1. Mega JL, Sabatine MS, Antman EM. Population and personalized medicine in the modern era. JAMA. 2014; 312(19): 1969-70.

2. Borkan J, Reis S, Steinmetz D, and Medalie JH. Patients and Doctors. Life changing stories from primary care. The University of Wisconsin Press. Madison, WI. 1999.

3. Yancey Philip. What's so amazing about grace? Zondervan Publishing House. Grand Rapids, MI. 1997.

## Crump, WJ. What Role Is Left For The Modern Doctor? Journal of Kentucky Medical Association. January 2015; (113): 25-27.

When I had the privilege of writing my first editorial for our journal five years ago, I had no idea that I would be writing my last one so soon. The needs of the modern medical association have changed dramatically during that short time period, and the idea of the old-fashioned state scientific journal seems quaint now. I do still hope that some entity will take on the task of publishing the work of our young academics, students, and residents as they test the waters of scientific writing. Our journal was an important vehicle for studies of local and regional medical issues, from opioid overdoses to pediatric head trauma. I trust the leadership of our association to find a new vehicle for communicating information on these important regional issues.

As I reflected on what to say in this last editorial, it seems that an historical perspective might be useful. My children know and my students have learned that I really believe that those who ignore history are doomed to repeat the mistakes of the past. By the way, I think with knowing history we still repeat most of the past mistakes, we just recognize them as they happen. A recently published medical history forms a good backdrop for this editorial. Written by a Baltimore historian, it chronicles the rise and fall of the perception of physicians in America from the glory days of colonial times beginning in 1620 to the "shambles" of American medicine in 1850 (1).

In colonial times physicians were held in high esteem despite having very few effective therapies. Blood-letting and purging were routine among orthodox physicians, but these were used in moderation. Mortality rates were high, but lower than what the new immigrants were accustomed to in Europe. Dispersed rural living and survival from previous old-country infections limited the effects of epidemics (except on the natives) and abundant food and game made life expectancy better than in Europe. And the quality of life was remarkable in the unspoiled wilderness. Folk healers including both African immigrant obeah and Native American shaman were also held in high esteem, and their use of roots and herbs were just as effective with less toxicity than those of the orthodox physicians.

Although orthodox physicians in Europe were gaining a reputation for being mercenaries and losing touch with their patients in the 1700s, this didn't begin in America until the early 1800s. It became clear that as Americans moved into cities and suffered massive epidemics of cholera, yellow fever, typhus, and other clustered infections, orthodox medicine had little to offer. "Sectarians" including purveyors of patent medicines, folk empiricism, homeopathy, hydrotherapy, mesmerism, and others seemed to get comparable outcomes with less toxicity. And the orthodox American physician held to the truth that Americans were so fundamentally different from Europeans that when the germ theory and aseptic practices were accepted in Europe, they were held in utter disdain by American medical leaders almost until the Flexner revolution and the rise of scientific medical training.

The historian attributes the success of both orthodox medicine and all the sectarians to an elaborate placebo effect. The air of authority and power, along with a bit of ritual, augmented the patient's own sincere hope that the healer could help him regain control of his life. When the rise of cities rendered the orthodox physician helpless, the sectarians stepped in. It is instructive to note what the orthodox physicians did in response. They accelerated their traditional methods: more heroic blood-letting and purging, higher doses of mercurials to the point of poisoning, all to try to reassert their preeminence. It is my sincere hope that we do not repeat that mistake.

It was not until the rise of true science in medicine in the early 1900s that a patient had more than a 50/50 chance of coming away from a doctor's visit any better than they entered. Vaccines and antibiotics, along with clean water and refrigeration, resulted in falling mortality rates. The Halcyon period for American physicians had begun, and their esteem steadily rose into the latter part of the twentieth century. The explosion of technology allowed us to see into every orifice, image the mysteries inside the body, and make real advances in medical and surgical treatment of most acute illnesses. Subspecialties emerged, and family doctors simply did the best they could directing medical traffic, even resulting in that terrible term of the 1980s and 90s, the gatekeeper.

As the millennium turned, something happened. Americans realized that we could not afford what we had constructed, and for the first time, the destructive potential of leading edge medicine was discovered. Just like the mercurials of the 1840s, more is not better. And the chronic, incurable diseases did not respond to new medicines like the older, acute ones did. Rediscovery of the value of a healthy lifestyle, risk factor management, and personal responsibility for one's health were not to be found in a pill bottle. Perhaps an historian or two are among the brave souls in national medical organizations who are now recommending that less intervention may actually not just be cheaper, but better for our patients (2).

So when my students read this editorial, what do I hope they will learn? In my humble opinion, it is not the air of authority that makes the "doctor as drug" so effective (3). Although I enjoy a bit of ritual as much as the next person, that's not it either. What made the orthodox physicians and then the sectarians, and then in turn the orthodox physicians again so effective was and is the relationship of the healer with the healed.

# FINDING MEANING IN WORK

As I have shared in these pages previously, Brody has summarized the three things that healers in all cultures do (4):

1. Provide a meaningful explanation for the illness
2. Express care and concern
3. Manage the possibility of mastery and control over the illness or its symptoms

And Brody again:

"The centrality of relationship as a way of both knowing and healing in primary care brings us back again to the importance of local knowledge. One forms relationships not with abstractions, but with specific people, families, and communities. ... even caring physicians dedicated to these relationships may fail, but physicians neglectful or dismissive of these relationships will almost certainly fail." Is it any wonder that our current medical system in America fails so many of us?

And from my favorite physician and priest (5):

"The human body is the place where human life and human love happen. The crafts of medicine, nursing, dentistry and all the other healing arts require at least two human bodies-that of the healer and that of the one who is healed. It is in human bodies that the spirit of God transforms the air we merely breathe into the grace of God that touches every cell in our mortal bodies, forms any words of Good News we will ever proclaim, and moves us to works of charity and worship."

So what should our association do to ensure that we have a role in the future of American medicine? As we are assailed from all sides from payers, government, and sectarians, I ask that you work to save our professional role. More procedures and more specialization are not necessarily better. Spend your resources strengthening the relationship of healer with the healed. What transpires in the best of medical care can simply not be accomplished by an anonymous "provider." When I'm in the mall and I overhear one of my patients lean over and say to their child "that's our doctor!" I know that there is hope.

Comments appreciated at bill.crump@bhsi.com

## References

1. Breslaw EG. Lotions, potions, pills, and magic: Health care in early America. New York University Press. New York. 2012.

2. The "Top 5" Lists in Primary Care: Meeting the Responsibility of Professionalism. Arch Intern Med. 2011;171(15):1385-1390.

3. Balint, Michael. The Doctor, His Patient and the Illness. Churchill Livingstone, 2000.

4. Borkan J, Reis S, Steinmetz D, and Medalie JH. Patients and Doctors. Life changing stories from primary care. The University of Wisconsin Press. Madison, WI. 1999.

5. Sulmasy DP. A Balm for Gilead. Washington, D.C. Georgetown University Press. 2006.

# MEDICAL SUPPORT TO INPATIENT PSYCHIATRY UNIT, 2006-2021

## CLINICAL STORIES

*Another inflection point in Dr. Crump's career came as he stepped down as journal editor and became the medical support to a locked inpatient psychiatry unit. The geriatric patients were medically complex, and the younger patients all had the saddest stories. Of the time, Dr. Crump says that before this he didn't realize just how often humans do terrible things to each other. So while important issues of the day continued to be addressed in his essays, he wrote more about the stories he heard from patients on the Psych unit. Two follow here.*

**Crump WJ. But doc, what if I can't die? The Journal of the Kentucky Academy of Family Physicians. Winter 2017;88:18**

One of my responsibilities is medical support to our behavioral health inpatient locked unit. Many of the stories are truly touching, but one will stick with me for a while. I went in to do the initial history and physical on a 68-year-old man who had been admitted for delusions. He had many medical problems, and had been admitted to inpatient psychiatric facilities previously. He was agitated, and I had already heard from the hall him say to the nurse "You just don't understand, you don't understand."

I introduced myself and explained my role as the medical doctor and asked if it was okay to speak with him a bit and do a brief physical exam. He reluctantly agreed. I always begin with "Please, tell me why you think you are here." His eyes blazed and then filled with tears. "Doc, I did some really terrible things when I was young. They are so bad that I don't feel that I can be forgiven. I think we are near the end of times and I am really, really scared. I feel that because of what I did that I will be left on earth forever, unable to die. Others will go on to their eternal reward but I will have to stay on earth forever, dealing with the pain and shame every day."

Caught more than a little off guard, I tried my usual "You know, when our thoughts are all mixed up sometimes things seem much worse than they actually are. Perhaps after we get your medicines straight these ideas won't seem so real."

As he turned away from me, he said "They couldn't get rid of these ideas at the state hospital no matter what." Again I tried to give a dose of hope, saying that we could talk again later when he felt more like talking. As I left the room, he turned towards me, and with blazing eyes again said, "But Doc, what if I'm right?"

The medication nurse was behind me coming into the room, and as I tried again to reassure him, he turned away and covered his head with the covers. The remainder of that day and into the night as I tried to fall asleep I continued to think of this patient. His fate as he understood it, did in fact, seem hopeless and terrifying.

Every day as I came into the unit and passed the area where he was eating breakfast with other patients, I would pause and make eye contact. Each day he would shake his head and nonverbally make it clear that he did not want to talk now. The psychiatrists worked their magic with atypical concoctions and he became less and less agitated. He told the nurses some pretty fantastical things that he might have done when he was young, but he was not interested in talking to me about any of these things.

Near the end of his almost 2 week admission, I saw that he was in his room alone and appeared alert. He seemed willing to talk, so I brought up the idea again. He said he still felt like he was to be punished at the end of times, but the thought was not quite as intrusive now.

Feeling that a doctor's number one responsibility is dispensing hope, I tried again. He was not interested in talking about what he did, but was interested in talking about God. I took a chance and suggested to him that God as I understood him was a forgiving God. Again the patient said that he could not imagine that anyone at any time could forgive him. I took another chance and said "I want you to know that right now I forgive you." I took his hands and tears welled up at his eyes again. He mumbled a thank you, and turned again, covering his head with the bedcovers.

The day prior to his discharge, as I walked through the breakfast area, he smiled warmly at me. But then he quickly looked away, appearing embarrassed. I don't know exactly what happened with him, except that he did go home to live with his wife, at least for a while. I think about him often.

I also wonder if I crossed al line, sharing my own faith with someone so vulnerable. And how could I be so arrogant that I would have the power of forgiveness?

Somehow, as I reflect on this interaction, it seems to have been the most important thing that I may have done that day. Healing goes both ways, and I never want to miss an opportunity.

## Crump, WJ. Those kids are rotten. The Journal of the Kentucky Academy of Family Physicians. 2018:90 (Spring):28

One of my current missions is to try to assist medical students and residents as they develop their professional identity. My goal is to make them a little less cynical. My favorite definition of a cynic is someone who cannot imagine anyone else being motivated by anything but self-interest. I also wish to inoculate them against severe burn out. The definition of burn out that I like the best is that it is a dislocation between what you thought you would be doing and what you actually end up doing. Another favorite description is that burn out is "erosion of the soul" that leads to ill health, depression, dissociation from important relationships and a downward spiral of worsening cynicism.

One of the exercises I do with my learners is to have them recall a situation where they clearly had one opinion and understanding of a patient that was dramatically different once the "rest of the story" was known. I use a short reflective video to get them started thinking, and then have them actually draw a comic with word balloons over the sketched characters, describing their understanding of the before and after versions of the patient stories.

As I did this comic drawing exercise myself, I recalled three women who I had seen recently in my role as medical support of our inpatient behavioral health unit, all admitted to the hospital for suicidal ideation, none on the unit at the same time. All three were angry with the world and each had new superficial linear lacerations on their arms that spoke to the need to feel something.

When taking their social and family history, each really focused on the disrespect shown them by their biological children, all teenagers. When I also asked as I always do about contraception, each said emphatically "Don't need any." So as always, I responded "So you're not having sexual intercourse?" Each responded negatively with some version of "Never again." All three of the women reported having current female partners.

I am often within earshot as the unit group sessions begin, and I overheard each of these women very angrily telling others about their kids. One said that she couldn't care less about her kids, and another said she didn't give a s - - - what happened to her kids. Each used some version of calling them "rotten," and each didn't care if she never saw them again.

So I made some assumptions about these women. The new partners were part of the household now, and I could imagine that unruly teenagers might not be entirely sensitive to their current situation and this behavior might actually make them feel more disconnected and hopeless.

None of the three stayed in the unit long enough for me to get to know them better. It was only in talking with the staff later that I discovered "the rest of the story." The story each patient told, confirmed by other family members, was that these children were the result of repeated rapes. One was by a step-father, one by an uncle, and one, especially troubling, was by her biological father.

These, and so many other stories from everyday practice, continually cause me to reflect and reconsider many assumptions. Humans can do bad things to each other, and my job is still to try to dispense hope every chance I get. Maybe by listening empathetically, our staff helped these women in some small way. Maybe each will share more in time with their outpatient therapist now that each has revealed it to the behavioral health staff. Some wounds don't begin to heal until the scab is off, I guess. And maybe the next time a physician sets aside cynicism and approaches them with genuine empathy, they will receive some solace. At least, that's my hope.

# COVID 2020-

*The next inflection was earth-shaking. An unusual pneumonia was first reported in China, and then cases began popping up on the American coasts. Dr. Crump recalls his son calling him from his home 3000 miles away and asking if he should be concerned because of his mild asthma. Dr. Crump responded that he expected this new illness to act like influenza, and if his son avoided people with active symptoms, all should be well. The tsunami of a pandemic crushed such thoughts. Asymptomatic infected individuals could transmit this terrible disease that had almost 10 times the mortality rate of influenza. Nothing would be the same. Dr. Crump and many other health care workers now worried about their own safety. He reports that not since the days of triple-gloving for procedures in patients at high risk for AIDs in the last century did each day present a health threat to him. As a form of therapy, again Dr. Crump wrote the following essays.*

## Crump, WJ. Covid 66: Are we too old for this? J Regional Med Campuses 2020 3(1)

As I drove in to make weekend rounds at our hospital, I noticed a buzzard circling above. It gave me pause. Well, I thought, at least it's just one buzzard. This whole social distancing thing has shaken me to my core.

As I passed my 65th birthday and watched all the subspecialists around me retire, I really had to stop and think what I would do if I no longer saw patients. And then I realized that at 65 our hospital bylaws said I could stop taking hospital night call. Fewer nighttime awakenings seemed like a good idea after 22 years of 24 /7 call backing up our residents' deliveries. But it slowly dawned on me that if I stopped taking night call and with younger faculty now available, it didn't seem reasonable for me to do daytime deliveries and ask them to do those at night. With that, a part of me that had been so integral stopped as well. I still oversee prenatal care with the residents, but have stopped doing deliveries. Life was less complicated, and I felt more rested and able to give my daytime work my full attention.

And then this confounded virus. Initially the CDC said that high-risk groups were older age and underlying conditions. I heard this three times from the same NIH official in the same day. Then somehow over the next few days their recommendations changed from "and" to "or". Suddenly, those of us with gray hair and perhaps some wisdom to share become at risk by doing what we've done every day for almost 40 years.

As we wait to see if the plague strikes our small regional hospital, disappointment is the reigning theme. I was scheduled to receive a national medical education award for our campus at the meeting in my hometown of Savannah. Family could attend and it seemed like a nice inflection point in my career. On the same weekend I could see my granddaughter play soccer in a tournament that is worthy of her Olympic development team skills. I could visit with the family and walk through the Cathedral, the squares downtown, and all of the places that made me who I am.

Meeting canceled, travel advisory for anyone my age, trip canceled, and disappointment. As we all struggle to decide what parts of medical education should still continue and whether we could possibly have any resident or medical student conferences with 6 feet between each learner, it suddenly dawned on me that I may be at risk in my own hospital.

I provide medical support for our inpatient geriatric behavioral health unit. What should I do the next time I'm called about a patient with fever and a cough? I could do a lot of the evaluation by video, but I'm just old-fashioned enough to need auscultation to help me make decisions. Although I used telemedicine auscultation 25 years ago with NASA, there's no quick way to set it up in our small hospital. And then there's the experience I had this morning. A woman just a few years older than I had been admitted for worsening dementia and some verbal aggression.

As I examined her, she ruminated with wild eyes on who would put her in such a place and asked me every few seconds how she could get out. No verbal reassurance worked, but when I just held her hand and told her how much we cared and how her family had entrusted her to our care, she visibly relaxed. There is no way we could have gotten to that first step of healing by video.

For those of us over 60 but still in good health and thrilled every day to see patients and interact with learners, what do we do? There are no clear guidelines. As I often do, I harken back to my mentor Dr. Gayle Stephens, who was one of the founding fathers of family medicine. Paraphrasing the central tenet of his philosophy: the definition of a family doctor is one who cannot ignore any issue brought to him by his patient.

I am going to find a way to get through this without losing who I am. And buzzards be damned.

## A VISIT TO THE CATHEDRAL
## MARCH 15, 2020

Covid 19 did something nothing else has done. This grown up good Catholic boy didn't attend mass today. I just watched the most moving livestream of morning mass from the Cathedral of Saint John the Baptist in Savannah. I was struck with the visual beauty, especially since it was mostly shown from the choir loft, a vantage point I have not seen since I was in a citywide parochial school choir singing at Holy Thursday services and funerals.

I was also struck with what was missing. As we older physicians try to find a way to serve our patients at a distance during this pandemic through the magic of telemedicine, video can only do so much. The smell of the incense and the feel of the organ within the pit of your stomach were missing. And the damp warmth of that old revered building and how even the sound of the choir seems to reverberate more in your bones than in your ears: missing.

Also missing was how one can gain a new perspective in person by just turning your head a bit. The light coming through the gorgeous stained glass windows changes the colors and the depth of what you see around you based on just that small change of viewing angle. And at communion time, I couldn't take the host within me, bringing back memories from childhood sensations of that dry sticky wafer that assured me that the Lord was now truly within me. And, on the way out after mass, not feeling the cool hard sensation of the marble as your knee touched it as you began your exit with genuflection.

Then I noticed things that were missing even with just the visual experience. The baptismal font had no water. There were small clusters of people who share a household, probably. There was about 6 feet between the clusters, something that would not be possible given the usual attendance Sunday at the Cathedral in Savannah. There was no handshake during the expression of peace, in fact no communal expression of peace at all. What was also striking is that several couples kissed anyway after the priest offered his expression of peace, as they had every Sunday. And the priest co-celebrant was within 6 feet of the celebrant as were the altar boys bringing up the book to be read and moving the incense back-and-forth. There was no wiping off of any of these sacred surfaces.

What have I missed and what are we missing? On my morning hospital rounds when the wild eyed elder who is convinced that she is being held against her will refused to be comforted by words, she seemed to have some peace when I just held her hand. How real is the value of human presence and human touch, with a bit of the Blessed thrown in. I need to go to mass in person in that Cathedral again. Soon.

## TIMELESS
## APRIL, 2020

This must be what retirement feels like. After almost 40 years of doing things by the clock, the need to know what time it is seems superfluous.

In my 20s and 30s, I fought for the first operative case of the morning slot so that I could actually start on time, and still get to the office on time. In the office, I pushed to get through on time so that I could make it to noon conference on time. In the afternoon, knowing that I still needed to make quick afternoon hospital rounds, I struggled to stay on time so that I could get home before my kids went to bed.

Then for the last 20 years or so, I have had a dean role, more education commitments, and slightly fewer clinical. Then it was a question of getting through with the late morning meeting in time to get to noon conference. And in the slots where I was precepting residents in their office, it was a push to finish seeing the new admissions in the morning while still getting there to be with the residents by nine. Then in the afternoon, it was managing the inevitable urgent student issues in time to get home before the latest of the steady stream of foster babies in our house went to bed.

My Catholic upbringing drove me to try to do everything on time. There was always a nun in full habit sitting (figuratively) on my shoulder whispering that being on time was showing respect. This all made me feel useful and productive.

Then COVID-19 happened. All group-teaching sessions were canceled. Students were required to leave any clinical contact. The hospital system within which we work requires almost all administrative workers to work from home. My small education wing that usually bustles with my staff making schedules and all of us working together to solve student problems goes quiet. A steady stream of students through our coordinator's office with an excuse to get chocolate from the jar on her desk (but really just there to let her mother them), stopped.

Even weekends are different. No more pushing to finish morning hospital rounds in time to pick up a grandchild and spend that precious time with each on a rotating basis every Saturday morning. And no more being sure I had set up things to record the key football or basketball game of the day so that after the time with the grandchildren I could settle down and do my third most favorite thing in the world.

And on Sundays, it was a matter of timing when I arrived at the hospital so I could get all the new admissions and acute problems dealt with in time to get to 10:30 mass and still get my favorite pew.

I really did believe it was the end of the world when the SEC basketball tournament was canceled. But that was only the beginning: all sports canceled, church services suspended.

What am I to do? It still bothers me not to know exactly what time it is very frequently, but there is no schedule. Even though still adapting to daylight savings time, the sun rises and sets at its usual time. I seem to get hungry and sleepy at the usual times. But there is no order to anything else.

If this is like retirement and I have paid all my dues along the way, I want my money back. How can one feel productive without a schedule? I think I will have to learn the answer to that. At least for now.

*Most of 2020 was a virtual blur, with zoom meetings, telemedicine patient visits, and remote lectures. In early summer 2021, vaccinations were widely available and the risk seemed much less. This was that magic window before the Delta variant surged later in summer and then the Omicron variant in the late fall. Dr. Crump reports that this window provided a glimmer of hope, prompting him to write the following essay that was published in his home parish bulletin.*

## COMING HOME
## JUNE, 2021

Why did I choose today to return to church in person? Maybe it was because I woke up with a migraine and couldn't spend my Sunday morning working on my book about Savannah's medical history as I had for months. I have to admit that having this time each week to write has been a source of renewal, and I could watch mass recorded later after my muse had gone quiet.

I can't really say it was because of the bishop's change allowing return in person. I'm just enough of a child of the 60s that, while I listen to church leadership, I make my own decisions. Was it to receive the Father's Day blessing in person? I have enough faith to believe that God's blessing can traverse cyber space and reach me, but it's just not the same.

Was it to see the members of my parish in person? Babies have been born and are entering early toddler stage since I last went in person. This includes at least one whose mother I saw grow up in our church. For whatever reason I got out my church shoes that I haven't worn in 15 months and made sure I got there early enough to back into my parking place. I drove a little slower up the hill than usual. I passed the school and had to pause a bit to consider my 12 years of Catholic schooling in Savannah. Then passing the parish hall, I remembered my daughter's wedding reception there as the last time that all four of my children were in the same place at the same time.

# FINDING MEANING IN WORK

It seemed a little strange walking towards the church and I had another real surprise. For a moment, I could not remember how to put my phone on vibrate. I had not done this in the 15 months away from my church. I also felt entirely differently. For almost 5 years, I was the medical support to our inpatient psychiatry unit. That meant quick early morning rounds on both Saturday and Sunday to be sure the physical needs of these precious souls were being attended to. This usually meant that I rushed to get into church on time, and had to be available by text to the nurses who were still trying to figure out the recommendations I left for them as I hurried out of the unit.

But this time, I was no longer in that role. I'm still teaching medical students and residents how to deliver healthy babies and I'm still staffing our cardiovascular screening efforts in local churches and food banks and covering our free clinic. But this morning, as on many other mornings recently, I was not rushed.

Still considering all that as I walked in, Father Carl's bright broad smile made me feel comfortable again. It was still strange not to shake his hand, but it was obvious that he was almost as happy to see me as I was to see him in person. Many others greeted me warmly. There were those who knew me in my professional doctor role and others who taught my kids in school or just seemed genuinely interested in what was going on in my life. It felt like home. I had attended virtually every Sunday, but it just wasn't the same.

When in-person services were stopped completely and our church was not yet equipped for live streaming, I connected to the live stream of the Cathedral in my hometown of Savannah. I wrote an essay on that experience that many found interesting, and rereading it now creates a perspective for my return to my home church today.

I didn't remember the church being that cool, and it felt good in the heat of today. And in the key part of the mass where you would expect the Spirit to be moving, there was that cracking sound made by the wind across the roofing tiles on this Church built "in the round" typical of the 1970s. Missing from the comparison to the cathedral was the resounding feeling in your gut of the organ in the choir loft where I spent many childhood hours practicing for Holy Thursday mass. But today here was a bright crisp guitar that brought me back to the church I attended in college at the University of Georgia. The folk style given to the traditional hymns again made me feel right at home.

Then there was the reading from the book of Job when God spoke from the storm and shut the doors of the sea saying, "thus far shall you come but no farther, and here shall your proud waves be stilled!" How many of us over the last 15 months could identify with Job?

And many of us have found solace in Psalm 103. Indeed "the Lord is kind and merciful." Next in Paul's letter to the Corinthians, he reassured us all that we didn't have to know Christ according to the flesh to be a full-fledged Christian and the old things have passed away and behold new things have come. Then Mark's account of the storm on the Sea of Galilee is more reassurance. I grew up around open sounds and ocean, and more than once got caught out in a boat too small in seas too rough, and used the prayer skills well that the nuns taught me.

I could always hear Father Carl's sermon clearly in the live stream, but the volume and brilliance of the sound in the church brought this Gospel story home in a more tangible way. What a reassuring thought. When things get out of hand, all we have to do is wake Jesus up. I couldn't help but consider that our parish was in stormy seas before Jesus woke up and sent us Father Carl: Now a congregation that is slowly growing, a childcare center that is flourishing, and a Catholic school that is now becoming the force that it should be.

But now the main event. In my essay about going to the Cathedral as a schoolboy, I described how the sensation of the host on your tongue is inextricably bound to the mystery of the true presence in the Eucharist. I had missed this. It was almost as if the person choosing the communion song knew what I needed. I did need the bread of life.

The blessing for fathers was touching and I did feel ready to go in peace when the mass was ended. The sending song said it well. You are higher than all of our questions, and you are deeper than all of our needs.

## FINDING MEANING IN WORK

So why did I choose today to return to church in person? Because I needed it, which is what I said in text to each of my children who wished me happy Father's Day. And in the words of the song for the preparation of the gifts, "Here I am Lord."

*During the late fall of 2021, the Omicron variant ravaged Dr. Crump's community, with largely the unvaccinated dying again in the local ICU. Sharing the frustration felt by most physicians, he responded to a request from the state journal for pieces concerning vaccine denial. As he often did, he reflected using an historical perspective.*

**Crump WJ. Emergency Use: A Revolutionary concept. Journal of the Kentucky Academy of Family Physicians. 2021;52:30**

General Washington saw it as a sign of weakness
And bore the scars

It was still experimental and strange it seemed
A simple scratch to protect an army?

Worth a try if hidden from enemy prying eyes
But at Valley Forge a last resort in full view

Masks not even a thought
And quarantine a reverse miasma

Psalm 91 says not to fear
Angels won't allow you to strike your foot upon a stone

But was it an angel of fear who guided Jenner?
The father of our country would say surely not.

During the critical part of the revolutionary war, Washington discovered that many of the British soldiers had been exposed to smallpox as children and therefore were immune. He realized that his forces were being decimated by this infection, as many of the colonists had not had previous exposure. Washington himself had contracted the disease in Barbados 25 years earlier, leaving him with a small scar on his nose. Quarantine was known to be effective, but was very unpopular and simply could not be enforced in tightly packed encampments. The irritation of quarantine was confounded by the prevailing concept at the time that plagues were spread by a cloud of evil termed a miasma. Variolation was established almost 20 years before Edward Jenner's landmark paper showing that inoculation with cowpox could prevent smallpox. The procedure during the time of Valley Forge required taking a small amount of exudate from a smallpox lesion and placing it in a scratch on the soldier's arm. The result was a very mild illness but sometimes quarantine was still suggested. Reports from the time show that Washington believed that if the enemy knew this process was going on with his army, they would know to attack while the Continentals were weakened. So he sent waves of his army away for this to occur, unknown to the enemy. In the truly desperate days of Valley Forge, he changed this policy to include variolation within the encampment.

The risk of this procedure for "emergency use" was that it would cause an outbreak within the encampment. In one of Washington's letters, he said he feared the disease more than the sword of the enemy. He accepted the risk, and the rest of the story, as they say, is truly history.

# DISCOVERING MY OWN PROFESSIONAL IDENTITY: FINDING MEANING IN WORK

*Dr. Crump describes these last 2 essays as the best descriptions of his professional life. He says these are a good way to end this description of a most interesting professional journey. For those interested in his life outside of traditional work, he suggests immersion into the <u>Healing Savannah</u> trilogy of books that he wrote and published in 2022.*

**Crump W.J. "Now Tell Me Again What You Are": A Family Doctor Reflects on the Importance of Context. Family Medicine. 2018 50(6):469-470. Copyright Society of Teachers of Family Medicine. Used by permission.**

When the third trainer asked me what I was it dawned on me that they might not get it. I was enduring the 16 hour training required for my third electronic medical record system in the last five years. As I had walked into the community college classroom building where I would undergo this indoctrination, the shiny chrome handrails and smooth slate tile floors were anything but welcoming. Things got off to a good start when I explained that I was a family doctor and we needed to start with building outpatient templates.

But when I explained that I deliver babies and I needed a delivery note and those orders, one trainer said " you can't do that." I paused and took a deep breath and thought about how many people have tried to tell me that over the last 35 years at multiple hospitals, I struggled to explain the concept of womb to tomb care. She said "that's great, but you can't do that the way templates are set up. You can only function in one context."

I thought about the metaphorical meaning of what she had just said. At some level I knew it was much more concrete. She sent me along to the "OB trainer" who had no problem setting me up for orders and delivery notes. She then said "so how about your postoperative orders?" I explained that although I did do C-sections for the first half of my career, I no longer do them because I am not needed to do that here. She said "oh, then you're a midwife?" I said no, but I would enjoy doing that for my next career. Again she just looked puzzled. After a lot of manipulations of mice and cursors, we agreed that she could set me up without having a C-section template and postoperative orders.

Then I explained that I did need the details of forceps and vacuum assisted deliveries within my note. You would've thought I had just spoken Russian. She said "you can't do that in this context." I was beginning to see a pattern. We worked our way through that with some phone calls to the man behind the curtain. Then I explained that I needed a newborn admission template and orders as well. The trainer let out what sounded like a groan and sent me along to the pediatrics room.

The pediatrics lady seemed really nice. She had a teddy bear on her mouse and offered me candy when we finished. That part went pretty well as it seemed I had gained some contextual competency. Then I explained that since I precept residents in their office I will need to be able to cosign their notes. With a look of disgust that didn't seem appropriate around kids, she pointed to the resident/ faculty area.

This part went pretty easily as he seemed to understand what I needed to do with the resident notes and orders but again "you can't do that in the context of your other templates." Then I explained that I provide medical support to our inpatient behavioral health unit, and needed a template for a consultant note. He frowned and decided to send me to the consultant training area.

The trainer said consultants have it really easy. There's just a standard note and only a few options and it's really simple. But again she explained that I could not do that in the context of the other templates. When I explained that I also see GYN patients in the main women's' center office and needed the orders for ultrasounds, mammography, and bone density, she said "well then you will have to talk to those people as well."

Down the hall with the smooth tile floors I went, wandering until I found the GYN room. The group was mostly quiet and I noticed most of them were my age. They seemed to have it pretty easy also. They had a few sets of standard orders and only a few templates and it seemed quite easy compared to everything else I do. And as I finished this training, I got the word again that I could not do that in the same context.

Near the end of the sessions, I finally was shown in to the man behind the curtain, and he explained that he would have to give me five separate contexts, and I would have to be very careful that I was in the correct one at all times. It was at this moment that I realized that Dr. Gayle Stephens had warned me of this almost 38 years ago as I began training in his residency in Birmingham. He explained that a family doctor is that modern medical healer who accepts the patient as he is, with no prerogative to ignore any complaint the sufferer brings, even if it appears non-medical on the surface1. As I walked back to my car, I had this image of these healers moving through multiple contexts like benevolent will-o- the- wisps, guiding their patients to safety. My challenge was to do what family doctors have always done. We simply go where we are needed, when we are needed, stepping through barriers when necessary.

I am told there are some good things about electronic medical records. Printed prescriptions are easier to read and their digital transmission works even better. The billing people are very happy with what I do, and someday I'm told that a population health approach can really happen from these records. Honestly, I think I might be in the retired population before that occurs.

Somehow this electronic medical record implementation shook me to my core and caused me to question if in fact I was what I thought I was all those years. But you know what? I am. I am a master of all contexts. I am my patient's doctor no matter the context. I am a family doctor. Bring on the next digital challenge!

Thank you, Dr. Stephens

## REFERENCES

1. Stephens G Gayle. The intellectual basis of Family Practice. 1982. Winter Publishing Co. Tucson AZ.

## Crump WJ. A Curious Reflection. Journal of Regional Medical Campuses

I recently received an invitation to provide a reflection at the beginning of our hospital medical staff meeting. Having attended these quarterly meetings in person with my colleagues while sharing an outstanding meal for almost 25 years, I had appreciated the short prayers and poems. We even had a Cappella rendition of an inspirational hymn one time. To engage attendees via zoom, I considered what a group of physicians and other providers who are giving up some of their evening for a meeting might appreciate. I decided that since we talk a lot about the Triple Aim in medicine but less about the importance of physician satisfaction as the fourth element that would be the topic of my 5 minute reflection.

My perspective on this issue is framed by the last eight years of our longitudinal study of changes in empathy and burnout among our medical students and residents (1-4). As we reviewed the literature, the definition for empathy that fits best for us is a true understanding of what it's like to be that patient. When a new diagnosis or a new medication or intervention is considered, how will it fit into the life of the individual in our exam room with us? In this sense empathy is a cognitive function and significantly different from the emotional aspects of feeling sympathy, which is something else. The literature is also clear that physicians with higher measured empathy not only have better patient outcomes and more satisfied patients, but they are happier themselves and report lower levels of burnout.

Studies of group physician practices show there are three elements that predict higher physician satisfaction and lower burnout. These are a personal sense of autonomy, agency, and meaning. Autonomy simply means that one has some influence over what goes on in their day-to-day practice. Agency means that one has influence over what the entire group does. Finding meaning in work is perhaps the most powerful factor in determining empathy and burnout.

The pursuit of meaning flourishes in the setting of empathy. The true practice of empathy requires continuing curiosity, as well as enough time with each patient to unleash that curiosity. As an attempt to widen the audience for this most important basic concept for patients and doctors, I had recently undertaken writing a trilogy of books using medical history as a vehicle (5). The physician energy invested in curiosity simply isn't captured by CPT codes or relative value units. Perhaps for this reason, the literature also shows that physician investment in curiosity wanes over time.

A landmark article was written by a general internist almost 25 years ago that highlights this. She says (6):

*… When I was a young attending at San Francisco General Hospital, morning rounds usually consisted of briefly going over the 15 to 20 patients admitted to the team the night before and then concentrating on the "interesting" ones. I was righteous and was determined to teach the house staff that there were no uninteresting patients, so I asked the resident to pick the dullest.*

*He chose an old woman admitted out of compassion because she had been evicted from her apartment and had nowhere else to go. She had no real medical history but was simply suffering from the depredations of antiquity and abandonment. I led the protesting group of house staff to her bedside. She was monosyllabic in her responses and gave a history of no substantive content. Nothing, it seemed, had ever really happened to her. She had lived a singularly unexciting life as a hotel maid. She could not even (or would not) tell stories of famous people caught in her hotel in awkward situations. I was getting desperate; it did seem that this woman was truly uninteresting. Finally, I asked her how long she had lived in San Francisco.*

*"Years and Years," she said*

*Was she here for the earthquake?*

*No, she came after.*

*Where did she come from?*

*Ireland.*

*When did she come?*

*1912.*

*Had she ever been to a hospital before?*

*Once.*

*How did that happen?*

*Well, she had broken her arm.*

*How had she broken her arm?*

*A trunk fell on it.*

*A trunk?*

*Yes.*

*What kind of trunk?*

*A steamer trunk.*

*How did that happen?*

*The boat lurched.*

*The boat?*

*The boat that was carrying her to America.*

*Why did the boat lurch?*

*It hit the iceberg.*

*Oh! What was the name of the boat?*

*The Titanic.*

She had been a steerage passenger on the Titanic when it hit the iceberg. She was injured, made it to the lifeboats, and was taken to a clinic on landing, where her broken arm was set. She now was no longer boring and immediately became an object of immense interest to the local newspapers and television stations – and the house staff...

I closed this brief reflection by saying that as we get back to in person human contact, hopefully soon without masks, my hope for us all is that we can rekindle our curiosity and find meaning in our work.

## *References*

1. Crump WJ, Ziegler CH, Fricker RS. A residency professional identity curriculum and a longitudinal measure of empathy in a community-based program. Journal of Regional Medical Campuses. 2018:1(4). doi: https://doi.org/10.24926/jrmc.v1i2.1292

2. Crump WJ, Fricker RS, Ziegler C. A closer look into empathy among medical students: The career eulogy as a lens. Marshall Journal of Medicine. 2021; 7(1): Article 6. doi: 10.33470/2379-9536.1317. Available at: https://mds.marshall.edu/mjm/vol7/iss1/6.

3. Crump WJ, Ziegler CH, Fricker RS. A longitudinal measure of medical student empathy at a regional campus: are we different? Could this be a valuable method for evaluating curriculum change? Journal of Regional Medical School Campuses. 2021; 4(1). doi: 10.24926/jrmc.v4i1.3475.

4. Crump WJ, Ziegler C, Fricker S. Empathy and Burnout During Residency: Which Changes First? Fam Med. 2022;54:640-643.

5. Crump WJ. Savannah's Bethesda. Healing for All. Self-published. July 20, 2022.

6. Fitzgerald F. Curiosity. 1999; Ann Int Med 130:70-72.

# APPENDIX: ORIGINAL PUBLICATIONS

Crump WJ, Ziegler C, Fricker S. Empathy and burnout during residency: Which changes first? Fam Med. 2022;54(8):640-643.

Leong, SL, Gillespie, CJ, Jones, B, Fancher, T, Coe, CL, Dodson, L, Hunsaker, M, Thompson, BM, Dempsey, A, Pallay, R, Crump, WJ, Cangiarella, JL. Accelerated 3-year MD pathway programs: Graduates' perspectives on education quality, the Learning environment, Residency readiness, debt, burnout, and career plans. Academic Medicine. 2022; 97(2):254-261.

Crump, WJ, Ziegler, CH, Fricker, RS. Do medical residents with rural upbringing show less decline in empathy during training? A report from a rural family medicine residency. Marshall Journal of Medicine. 2022; 8(1): Article 6.

Parker, SR, Crump WJ. Who really wants to be somebody's doctor? Journal of the Kentucky Academy of Family Physicians. 2022;53:28-29.

Doyle EC, Southall WR, Edmonson BS, Crump WJ. A student-directed community cardiovascular screening project at a regional campus. Journal of Regional Medical School Campuses. 2021; 4(4).

Crump WJ, Ziegler CH, Fricker RS. Does empathy really decline during residency training? A longitudinal look at changes in measured empathy in a community program. Journal of Regional Medical School Campuses. 2021; 4(4).

Crump WJ. Emergency Use: A Revolutionary concept. Journal of the Kentucky Academy of Family Physicians. 2021;52:30.

Beck AT, Cleaver LB, Fuqua JD, Clark KB, Nair RS, Hart EP, Bolinger RR, Crump WJ. A Teleneurology teaching service at a rural regional campus: An effective solution when specialty availability is limited. Journal of Regional Medical Campuses. 2021; 4(3).

Dodd B, Crump WJ. The real social history: the value of unhurried listening. Journal of the Kentucky Academy of Family Physicians. Winter 2021; 49:28-30.

Crump WJ, Nims, DM, Hatler DJ. Mr. Watson, come here I want to see you: one rural residency program's rapid pivot to telemedicine during the pandemic. Marshall Journal of Medicine. 2021; 7(2): Article 8.

Crump WJ, Ziegler, CH, Fricker, RS. A longitudinal measure of medical student empathy at a regional campus: are we different? Could this be a valuable method for evaluating curriculum change? Journal of Regional Medical School Campuses. 2021; 4(1).

Crump WJ, Fricker RS, Ziegler, C. A closer look into empathy among medical students: The career eulogy as a lens. Marshall Journal of Medicine. 2021; 7(1): Article 6.

Crump, WJ. Telemedicine: has the time really finally arrived? Journal of Rural Health. 2021; 37(1):156-157.

Fisher SM, Crump WJ. Stepping up to the plate: An unexpected leadership opportunity during the COVID-19 Pandemic. Journal of Regional Med Campuses. 2020; 3(3).

Holthouser AL, Farmer RW, Crump WJ, Shaw, MA. University of Louisville School of Medicine: Medical Education Program Highlights. Academic Medicine. 2020; 95(9): S192-S195.

Beck AT, Crump, WJ, Shah JJ. Neurology Telemedicine as Virtual Learning for Regional Medical Campuses. Journal of Regional Medical Campuses. 2020; 3(2).

Roby SL, Crump WJ, COVID 19: We can't go over it. We can't go under it. We've got to go through it. The Journal of the Kentucky Academy of Family Physicians., 2020;47 (Summer):16-18.

Crump WJ, Fricker RS, Crump-Rogers, A. A Career Eulogy Reflective Exercise: A View into Early Professional Identity Formation. Marshall Journal of Medicine 2020 6(2) Article 12.

Crump, WJ. Covid 66: Are we too old for this? J Regional Med Campuses 2020 3(1).

Crump WJ, Fricker RS, Crump AM. Professional identify formation among college premedical students: a glimpse into the looking glass using a Career Eulogy reflective exercise. J Regional Med Campuses. 2019:2(2).

Engelbrecht AB, Higdon RE, Marshall, HM, Parker SR, Shelton BS, Crump WJ. A brief exercise in narrative medicine for preclinical medical and premedical students: My Story. J of Regional Medical Campuses. 2019; 2(5).

Whittington CP, Crump WJ, Fricker, RS. An invitation to walk a mile in their shoes: a rural immersion experience for college pre-medical students. Journal of Regional Medical School Campuses. 2019;1(5).

Clark AR, Smith, JT, Tucker, CS, Travis EW, Crump WJ. In the eastern fields of Eden. Journal of Regional Medical School Campuses. 2019;1(5).

Crump AM, Jeter K, Mullins S, Shadoan A, Ziegler C, Crump WJ. Rural Medicine Realities: The Impact of Immersion on Urban-Based Medical Students. Journal of Rural Health. 2019; 35(1):42-48.

Crump WJ. A closer look at an ezetimibe discussion. The Journal of Family Practice. 2018: 67(11): 675-676.

Crump WJ, Ziegler CH, Fricker RS. A residency professional identity curriculum and a longitudinal measure of empathy in a community-based program. Journal of Regional Medical Campuses. 2018:1(4).

Crump W.J. "Now Tell Me Again What You Are": A Family Doctor Reflects on the Importance of Context. Family Medicine. 2018 50(6):469-470.

Crump WJ; Ziegler CH, Fricker, RS. Rural Medical Student Opinions About Rural Practice: Does Choice of College Make a Difference? Marshall Journal of Medicine. 2018: 4(3), Article 7.

Logan L, Severns, A, Crump WJ. Community assessment of cardiovascular risk: an application for rural Kentucky. The Journal of the Kentucky Academy of Family Physicians. 2017;89 (Winter):26-29.

Fazenbaker SC, Crump-Rogers, AM, Crump, WJ and Langston, L. The Impact of Neonatal Abstinence Syndrome: The View from a Rural Kentucky Hospital. Marshall Journal of Medicine. 2017:3(3), Article 10.

Crump WJ, Ziegler CH, Martin LJ, Fricker RS, Shaw, MA, Crump AM, Sawning S. Changes in rural affinity among rural medical students as they experience education in an urban setting. Marshall Journal of Medicine. 2017;2(1).

Crump B. Professional Identity Curriculum at the University of Louisville Trover Campus: Reflection and Meaning in Medical Education. The Journal of the Kentucky Academy of Family Physicians. Winter 2017;88:18.

Crump WJ, Weaver AD, Fricker RS, Crump, AM. (2016) Why Medical Students Choose Rural Clinical Campuses for Training: A Report from Two Campuses at Opposite Ends of The Commonwealth. Marshall Journal of Medicine. 2016; 2(4): 15.

Crump WJ, Fricker RS. Keeping Rural Medical Students Connected to their Roots: A "Home for the Holidays" Immersion Experience. Marshall Journal of Medicine. 2016; 2(1):8

Crump WJ, Fricker RS, Fisher SM, Nair RS. A Glimpse of the Transition of Care from Free Clinic to Medicaid. The Journal of the Kentucky Academy of Family Physicians. Winter 2016; 87:8-10.

Crump WJ, Fricker RS, Ziegler CH, Wiegman DL. Increasing the Rural Physician Workforce: A Potential Role for Small Rural Medical School Campuses. The Journal of Rural Health. 2016; 32(3):254-259.

Crump WJ, Fricker, RS. A Medical School Prematriculation Program for Rural Students: Staying Connected With Place, Cultivating a Special Connection With People. Teaching and Learning in Medicine. 2015; 27(4): 422-430.

Crump WJ, Jessup, Ashley. Early Experience with an Accelerated Medical School Track to Rural Practice. Journal of Kentucky Medical Association. 2015; 113: 55-57.

Crump WJ, Fricker RS, Ziegler CH, Wiegman DL. Seeking the Best Dose of Rural Experience: Comparison of Three Rural Pathways Programs at One Medical School. Journal of Kentucky Medical Association. 2015; 113: 5-15.

Crump WJ, Fricker RS, Flick, KF, Gerwe-Wickham K, Greenwell, K, Willen KL. A Rural Pathways Program for High School Students: Reinforcing a Sense of Place. Family Medicine. 2014; 46(9): 713-717.

Crump WJ, Fisher SM, Fricker RS. Community Service as Learning Laboratory: A Report of Six Years of a Rural Community-Academic Partnership. Journal of the Kentucky Medical Association. 2014; 122: 131-136.

Crump WJ, Fricker RS, Ziegler C, Wiegman DL, Rowland ML. Rural Track Training Based at a Small Regional Campus: Equivalency of Training, Residency Choice, and Practice Location of Graduates. Academic Medicine. 2013; 88(8): 1122-1128.

Crump WJ, Lang Joan, Fricker RS, Settle Megan, Lewis Amanda. Acceptability of fecal occult blood testing for colorectal cancer screening: A Community-Based Effort. Journal of the Kentucky Academy of Family Physicians. Autumn 2013; 20: 9-13.

Crump WJ, Wood RL, Dave S, Javaid Z. First Steps Toward a Patient Centered Medical Home in a Family Medicine Residency Practice: The Huddle. Journal of the Kentucky Academy of Family Physicians. Autumn 2013; 20: 18-22.

Crump WJ, Dave S, Javaid Z, Wood, RL. One Residency's Experience With Beginning the Transition to a Patient Centered Medical Home Model. Journal of the Kentucky Academy of Family Physicians. Summer 2013; 79: 15-18.

Crump WJ, Wiegman David L, Fricker RS. An Accelerated Track to Rural Practice: An Option to Complete Medical School in Three Years.

Journal of the Kentucky Academy of Family Physicians. Winter 2013; 78: 20-22.

Crump WJ, Miller KH, Fricker RS, Pradip P, Ostapchuck M. An innovative Technique for Faculty Development at a Rural Kentucky Clinical Campus. Journal of the Kentucky Medical Association. 2012; 110: 274-282.

Crump WJ Jr, Carter P, Crump WJ III. Prematriculation medical students as agents of change: The Change Assessment Project. Journal of the Kentucky Academy of Family Physicians. Spring 2011; 71: 9-12.

Crump WJ Jr, King MA, Matera EL, Crump WJ III. Experience with a medical student-directed free clinic: Patient, student, staff, and faculty perspectives. Journal of the Kentucky Medical Association. 2011; 109: 9-14.

Crump WJ, Fricker RS, Ziegler CH. Outcomes of a preclinical rural medicine elective at an urban medical school. Family Medicine. 2010; 42(10): 717-722.

Crump WJ, Fricker RS, Wiegman DL. A 10-year Evaluation of the Trover Campus: Lessons learned for addressing the need for more rural physicians. Journal of the Kentucky Medical Association. 2010; 108(5): 137-143.

Roby SL, Crump WJ, Fricker RS. Prenatal care access for low English proficiency women: a review of some barriers and the role of lay health volunteers as a partial solution. Journal of the Kentucky Medical Association. May 2010; 108: 270-273.

Crump WJ, Fricker RS, Wiegman DL. The role of a rural medical school campus in developing a sense of place: the first 10 years. Family Medicine. 2010; 42: 160-161.

Crump, WJ, Fricker, RS, Crump AM. Just what are pre-medical students thinking?: A report of the first 6 years of a pathways program. Journal of Rural Health. January 2010; 26(1): 97-99

Crump WJ, Fricker RS, Crump AM. James, T.E. Outcomes and cost savings of free clinic care. Journal of the Kentucky Medical Association. August 2006; 104(8): 340-343.

Crump WJ, Crump AM. A community-based colorectal cancer screening initiative. Journal of the Kentucky Academy of Family Physicians. Fall, 2005; 53: 4-5.

Crump WJ, Moore AC. Experience with a rural medicine elective for preclinical medical students at an urban medical school. Journal of the Kentucky Academy of Family Physicians. Winter 2004; 50(1): 9-14.

Crump WJ, Fricker S, Barnett D. A Sense of Place: Rural training at a regional medical school campus. Journal of Rural Health. January 2004; 20(1): 80-84.

Crump WJ, Wood RL, Crump SE. Continuity Maternity Care Training for Family Practice Residents: A Community Hospital Experience. Journal of the Kentucky Academy of Family Physicians. August 2003; 49(3): 10-12.

Crump WJ, Fricker S, Brown A. Coakley V. An innovative method for preparation for rural practice: The High School Rural Scholars Program. Journal of the Kentucky Medical Association. November 2002; 100(11): 499-504.

Crump WJ. The Trover campus in Madisonville: The western Kentucky commitment to training physicians for rural areas. Journal of the Kentucky Academy of Family Physicians. November 2001; 47(4): 9-12.

Crump WJ, McCall Luke, Phebus Carol, and England Leigh. The Rural Health Career Pipeline Program: Report of a Pilot Project Summer, 2000. Journal of the Kentucky Academy of Family Physicians. May 2001; 47(2): 16-18.

Crump WJ. Clinical Telemedicine: What is the value for the family physician? Louisville Medicine. September 2000; 48(4): 60-161.

Crump WJ, Privett JD and Kennedy ME. Videophone Telemedicine Use in a School-Based Clinic. Journal of the Kentucky Academy of Family Practice, February 2000; 6(1):15-16.

Brooks RW, Martin DA, Crump WJ, et al. Community Assessment Using the Key Informant Method: A Snapshot of Some Rural Communities from the Perspective of Community Leaders. Journal of the Kentucky Medical Association. January 2000; 98(4): 27-30.

Li KH, Tang RA, Oschner K, Koplos C, Grady J and Crump WJ. Telemedicine Screening of Glaucoma, Telemedicine Journal. November 1999; 5(3): 283-290.

Crump, WJ, and Bersch, RB. A practice-based rural health fellowship: an innovative approach to support for rural care. Texas Medicine. November 1999; 5(11): 2-77.

Todini, Carole R and Crump WJ. Building a Regional Clinical Campus: Experience with Preclinical Students. Family Medicine. January 1999; 1(1): 6-7.

Crump WJ, State-of-the-Art: Interactive Videoconferencing for community-based medical school experience. Louisville Medicine. 1998; 46(7): 341-345.

Crump WJ, Caskey JW and Ferrell BG. The Effect of a Remote Facilitator on Small-Group Problem Solving: Potential Uses of Two-Way Video Technology in Decentralized Medical Education. Teaching and Learning in Medicine. 1998; 10(3): 172-177.

Crump WJ, Kumar R, Orsak G and Pfeil T. A Field Trial of Two Telemedicine Camera Systems in a Family Practice. Archives of Family Medicine. 1998; 7(2): 174-176.

Crump WJ, Boisaubin E, and Camp L. The Community Continuity Experience: Generalist Training for Preclinical Medical Students. Texas Medicine. 1998; 94(3): 58-63.

Crump WJ, Becker M, Speer A, Thompson B, Wainwright M. Brief Individualized Teaching Skills Workshops for Community Faculty: A Multispecialty Approach. Family Medicine. April, 1997; 280.

Crump WJ, Tessen RJ and Montero AJ. The Department Without Walls: Acceptability, Cost, and Utilization of Interactive Video Technology. Archives of Family Medicine. 1997; 6: 273-278.

Crump WJ and Tessen, RJ. Communication in Integrated Practice networks: Using Interactive Video Technology to Build the Medical Office Without Walls. Texas Medicine. 1997; 93(3): 70-75.

Crump WJ, Kottke TE, Perednia DA, and Sanders JH. Is Telemedicine Ready for Prime Time? Patient Care. 1997; 31(3): 64-87.

Crump WJ, Levy BJ and Billica RD. A Field Trial of the NASA Telemedicine Instrument Pack in a Family Practice Telemedicine Testbed. Aviation, Space, and Environmental Medicine. 1996; 67(11): 1080-1085.

Crump WJ, Chambers DL and Bolt J. Initial Community Site Development For First- and Second-year Medical Students. Family Medicine. 1996; 28: 634-639.

Crump WJ, and Driscoll B. An Application of Telemedicine Technology for Otorhinolaryngology Diagnosis. Laryngoscope Journal. 1996; 106: 595-598.

Crump WJ and Pfeil T. A Telemedicine Primer For The Primary Care Physician: An Introduction To The Technology And An Overview Of The Literature. Archives of Family Medicine. 1995; 91(7): 62-67.

Crump WJ, Levy BJ and Spann SJ. The Medical School Without Walls: Who Will Be The Faculty? Texas Medicine. 1995; 91(7): 63-67

Crump WJ, Marquiss C, Pierce P, and Phelps TK. The decision to suggest screening lower gastrointestinal endoscopy: The effect of training. Family Medicine. 1991; 23(4): 267-274.

Crump WJ and Phelps TK. Teaching Lower Gastrointestinal Endoscopy: A Comparison of Family Medicine and Internal Medicine Residencies. Journal of American Board of Family Practice. 1991; 4(1): 1-4.

Crump WJ, Marquiss C, and Pierce P. A practice-based analysis of the impact of family physicians' cessation of obstetric care. Alabama Medicine. 1990; 59(12): 26-30.

Crump WJ. Oxytocin and the Induction of Labor: Use in a Network of Community Hospitals. Family Medicine. 1989; 21: 110-113.

Crump WJ. Status Report: Family Practice Obstetrics in Alabama—More Bad News. Alabama Medicine. May 1988; 47-49.

Crump WJ and Massengill P. Outpatient Consultations from a Family Practice Residency Program: Nine Years' Experience. Journal of American Board of Family Practice. 1988; 1: 154-166.

Crump WJ. Excessive Weight Gain and Pregnancy Outcome. Alabama Medicine. 1988; 57(9):19-26.

Crump WJ. Postdate Pregnancy in a Network of Community Hospitals: Management and Outcome. Journal of Family Practice. 1988; 26(1): 41-44.

Crump WJ. The Alabama Perinatal Outcome Project: Some Methodological Issues. Family Practice Research Journal. Fall 1987; 7(1): 3-11.

Crump WJ. Obstetrical Practice Style and Clinical Policy in Residency Training. Family Medicine. 1987; 19(5): 378-379.

Crump WJ. The Bishop Score and Labor Duration: A New Look. Southern Medicine Journal. 1987; 80(10): 1294-1295.

Banahan BF, Jr, Anderson RL, Banahan BF, III, and Crump WJ. Physicians' Evaluation of Their Moonlighting During Residency Training. Journal of Medical Education. April 1987; 62: 351-353.

Crump WJ and Redmond DB. A Survey of Family Physicians Providing Obstetrical Care. Alabama Medicine. April 1986; 26-27.

Crump WJ and Redmond DB. A Survey of Family Physicians Providing Obstetrical Care: A Preliminary Report. Alabama Medicine. March 1986; 39-40.

Bartlett E, Pegues HU, Shaffer CR, and Crump WJ. Health Hazard Appraisal in a Family Practice Center: An Exploratory Study. Journal of Community Health. Winter 1983; 9(2): 135-144.

Kochert G and Crump WJ. Reversal of Sexual Induction in Volvox carteri by Ultraviolet Irradiation and Removal of Sexual Pheromone. Gamete Research. 1979; 2:259.

Data JL, Gerber JG, Crump WJ, et al. The Prostaglandin System: A Role in Canine Baroreceptor Control of Renin Release. Circ Research. 1978; 42:454.

## TEXTBOOKS/CHAPTERS:

Crump W, O'Kelley S. Care of the Newborn. FP Essentials. American Academy of Family Physicians. August 2012; (399): 1-48.

Crump WJ. Depression. Monograph, Edition No. 171, Home Study Self-Assessment Program. Kansas City, MO.: American Academy of Family Physicians. 1993.

Schwiebert LP and Crump WJ. Dysuria in Females. Chapter for Ambulatory Medicine: Primary Care of Families. Appleton & Lange, 1993.

Crump WJ. Congestive Heart Failure. Monograph, Edition No. 153, Home Study Self-Assessment program. Kansas City, Mo.: American Academy of Family Physicians. February 1992.

Crump WJ. Reflux Esophagitis: Diagnosis, Pathophysiology, and Management. Primary Care. 1988; 15(1): 13-30.

## CLINICAL REVIEWS/CASE STUDIES:

Crump WJ. New guidelines for managing neonatal jaundice: A case-based report. Family Practice Recertification. July 2005; 27(7): 40-49.

Crump WJ. Prenatal screening for common genetic diseases: A cased-based report. Family Practice Recertification. October 2004; 26(10): 47-54.

Crump WJ. Management of Group B Strep colonization during pregnancy and delivery. The Core Content Review of Family Medicine. January 2003; 34(1): 34.

Crump, WJ. What should I tell this woman now about hormone replacement therapy? Family Practice Recertification. September 2002; 24(10): 14-19.

Crump WJ. Pregnancy and the depressed patient: A case-based report. Family Practice Recertification. April 2002; 24(4): 67-72.

Crump WJ. When the OB patient has suffered minor trauma. Family Practice Recertification. February 2002; 24(2): 49-55.

Crump WJ. The pregnant patient with chronic hypertension. Family Practice Recertification. December 2001; 23(14): 39-43.

Crump WJ. The patient with no prenatal care: Managing an infant whose mother used cocaine. Family Practice Recertification. July 2001; 23(9): 48-55.

Crump WJ. The patient with no prenatal care: Delivery and immediate postpartum course. Family Practice Recertification. June 2001; 23(8): 47-56.

Crump WJ. Managing adolescent sports head injuries: A case-based report. Family Practice Recertification. March 2001; 23(4): 27-33.

Crump WJ. The pregnant patient at risk for hepatitis. Family Practice Recertification. November 2000; 22(14): 49-61.

Crump WJ. The pregnant day-care worker: What are the infectious risks? Family Practice Recertification. September 2000; 22(11): 21-32.

Crump WJ. UTIs in pregnancy: A case-based report. Family Practice Recertification. September 1999; 21(10): 45-56.

Crump WJ and Aten LA. Hyperemesis, Hyperthyroidism, or Both? Journal of Family Practice. 1992; 35(4): 450-456.

Shearer B, McCann L, and Crump WJ. Grateful Med: Getting Started. Journal of American Board of Family Practice. 1989; 3(1).

Crump WJ. What the Courts Are Saying About Living Wills. Senior Patient. 1989; 1(2): 76-83.

Crump WJ. Helping Your Patient Prepare a Living Will. Senior Patient. 1989; 1(2): 85-92.

Shearer B, McCann L, and Crump WJ. A Primer for Users of Medical Bibliographic Databases. Journal of American Board of Family Practice. 1989; 2(3): 191-195.

Crump WJ. Current Use of the Papanicolaou Smear. Journal of American Board of Family Practice. 1988; 1(2).

Crump WJ. The Honeymoon Period in Non-Insulin Dependent Diabetes Mellitus. Journal of Family Practice. 1987; 25(1): 78-82.

Crump WJ and Smith CW. The Postdate Pregnancy: When to Wait, When to Induce Labor. Postgraduate Medicine. 1986; 80(5): 291-297.

Made in the USA
Columbia, SC
18 April 2023